BOB THE BATHROOM
SCALES, AND ME

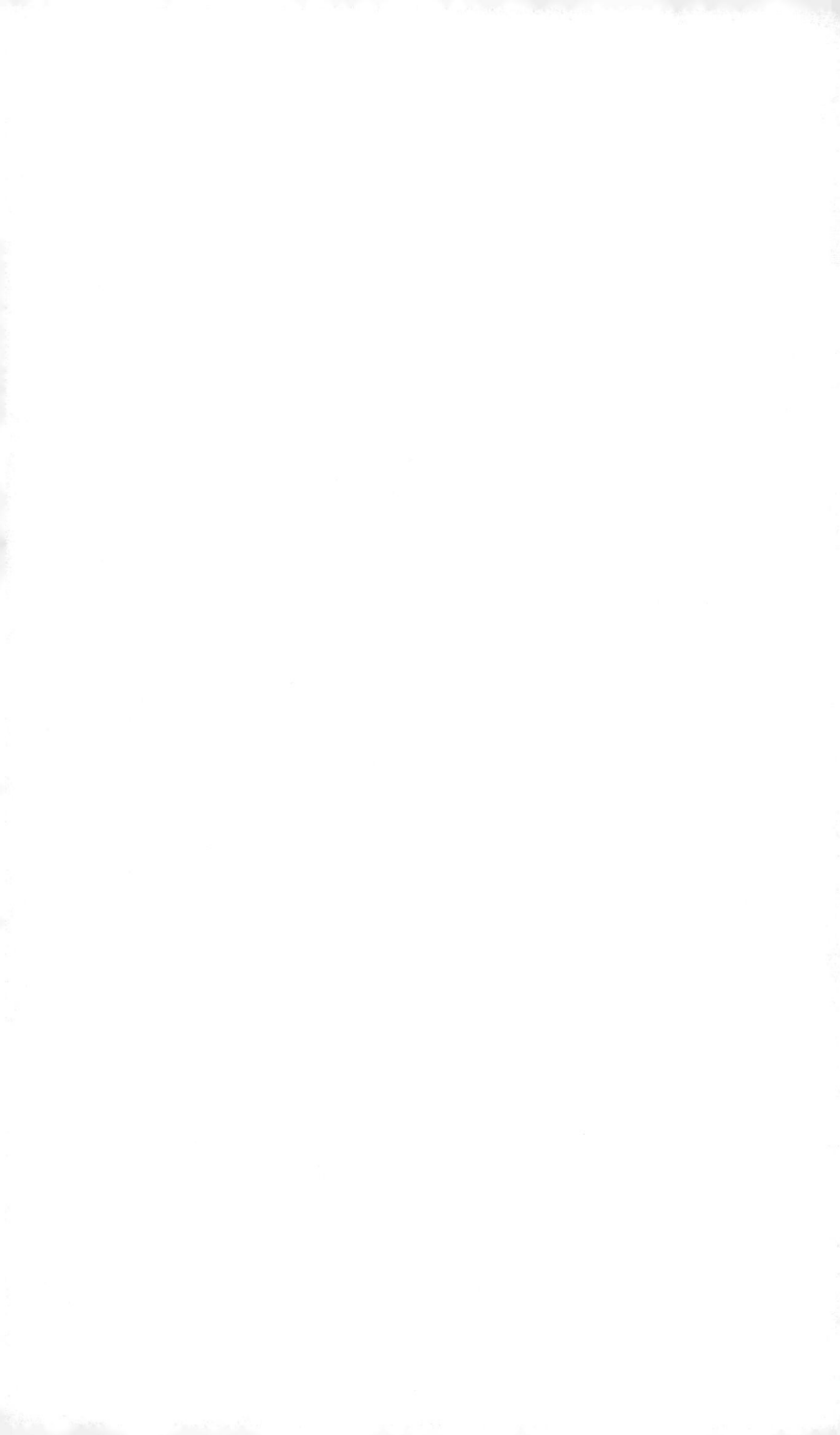

BOB THE BATHROOM SCALES, AND ME

Dena Valley

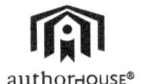

authorHOUSE®

AuthorHouse™ LLC
1663 Liberty Drive
Bloomington, IN 47403
www.authorhouse.com
Phone: 1-800-839-8640

Published by AuthorHouse   08/27/2013

ISBN: 978-1-4817-7786-5 (sc)
ISBN: 978-1-4817-7785-8 (e)

Registration Number: TXu 1-859-857

Contents

Many Thanks

My deepest gratitude to Nancy Goodman and Dave Ports for their invaluable assistance editing this book. And thanks to all my friends and family for their encouragement and help naming this book.

Remember the last scene in Casablanca at the airport where Humphrey Bogart and Claude Raines are walking away together and Bogart says, "I think this is the beginning of a beautiful friendship". That could be true here and the friendship would be with yourself.

Foreword

Good grief. My butt needs its own zip code! With a familiar numbness I head to the mall for larger size pants. Numb and semiconscious much of the time, this was my life.

How did this happen? It turns out it was effortless. Over the years I'd gained an average of less than two pounds a year. That was nothing . . . unless you are consistent like me and did it for more than 35 years. That is almost 20 pounds a decade and 70 pounds over the years. My 5'1" frame was now hauling around way too much weight. I discarded my scales some time back so I wouldn't have to face the truth. But when I went to buy pants there were a whole lot of X's on the label.

A few years back I began thinking that I'd really like to lose weight easily and naturally in a happy, healthy way. I knew I had to begin eating better and in a more satisfying way than the present way I was doing food. I knew I didn't want to count calories, carbs or fat grams ever again. Except for all those short times I'd gone on the latest diet I'd pretty much ignored my body.

I've been blessed with good health throughout my life but started gaining extra weight when I was about four years old. I spent my years in school trying to hide.

I didn't want people to see me nut of course they did. When a little boy I had a crush on called me fatso one day I wanted to die. About that time there was a popular song called "She's Too Fat For Me". I was certain it had been written just to torment me.

Society demands that we women look like what we see on television and magazines. Sometimes I get the feeling the world wants all women to be Parsley People . . . look very decorative on the outside but have no clue of our value on the inside.

My first diet was the grapefruit diet when I was twelve. Grapefruit was all I ate for a week. Since then I've been on hundreds of diets. My favorite for about a day and a half was a diet of wine and cheese. Yes, I actually read somewhere that it was an excellent diet.

PART I

The Seed

One day I told my daughter Heidi that I intended to do my best to stay away from negative thinking. I grew up with pretty positive thinkers but I could find myself in some very dark, depressed moods at times and could be very critical of myself and others. The new change in attitude proved to be the catalyst for a huge shift in my life.

About a month later I reread a book by Louise Hay called *You Can Heal Your Life*. It said that fear, anger, resentment and guilt did more harm in our lives than pretty much anything else. Then it said to look into a mirror and say "I love you". I'd done this many times before but this day was different, very different. I cried a torrent of tears and surrendered to grief there at the bathroom mirror. I could barely look at the mess before me. The feeling of guilt and shame came down on me hard that afternoon and it took me by surprise.

I'd always thought guilt was the least of my problems. Not so. It became totally clear that I felt wretchedly guilty for being a huge disappointment to my mom and dad (or so I thought), being a disgustingly weak parent and last but not least the betrayal and disappointment of letting myself down. Guilty, guilty, guilty. Through all those tears I had no idea my life would change.

The authentic me began to emerge and I began craving fresh fruits and vegetables. They had always been okay with me but now they were at the top of my grocery list. The four P's (Pasta, pastry, pop and processed products which for me meant TV dinners. no longer called to me. I haven't eaten pasta in months although I have nothing against it. It still tastes pleasant but it isn't important to me anymore.

I began consciously listening to my mind and body and that was totally new for me. I was a kid during World War II and my mom and dad felt terrible about the suffering in Europe, especially all those people starving. So they continually insisted I clean my plate so I wouldn't waste food. I also remember family gatherings where there was a small amount of food left in a serving dish. "Clean this up", whoever did the cooking would say, "I don't want to have to save that little bit." I often played garbage disposal during those times. I've carried that with me all my life. But now I remind myself I have choices now and I'm not a human garbage disposal.

I try to stay in tune to this because I know it's a big key for me. It's the hardest thing to do on this diet until you get used to it. We Americans usually just toss food down our throat. Have you ever watched a person eat snacks while watching TV? They are about 98% unaware of the amount of food consumed. And it is almost never raw vegetables they are feeding on.

The strange thing was that I changed almost the minute I stopped sobbing (which took me about three days). The wretched guilt I'd been wrapped in all those years began falling away and I found I just didn't have the same kind of energy on food. I eat anything I want whenever my stomach says to, but junk food and the four P's don't call to me now.

I think it's been the dawn of sanity. The resolve to stay away from negative thinking strengthened that. My mind did a lot of editing at first to stay away from those kind of thoughts but it gets easier. Strangely enough those two things seemed to be the true diet for me. Food was no longer the big enemy. Being critical and unforgiving were my two big issues.

I've thought a lot about how people seem to always be on a diet without any permanent success. We all have unhealed issues, and for me this planet is one big convalescent hospital. We are all here to help heal and be healed.

Some souls have the burden from birth of not being born the right sex. I know my mom wanted a girl badly. But the depression was dragging on and they already had a son. Those times must have been difficult for young marrieds. No wonder there were so many families with only one child.

Some children were physically or mentally abused during childhood. We blamed ourselves and that became our core belief. We labeled ourselves as failures, rejects, defective and guilty. We mistakenly took on all the shame, low self esteem, powerlessness and in my case sadness, and carried these feelings throughout our lives.

How can we expect to be successful at losing weight if we continue to believe that we are failures? I betrayed myself hundreds of times with food. Our core beliefs and self talk must change to be successful. And that can happen.

I just needed to pull my Get Out Of Jail Now card out of my back pocket. What that required was to take a hard look at the emotions you had when you first began to put on extra weight and give up stories like: I have a slow metabolism, or I've tried everything and nothing works, or I just like pie and cookies too much, or It's just too difficult while cooking for a family, or it's just too late for me. Another story I had in my head was I'm not good at this mind stuff. It doesn't work for me. It was time to dump all that, and begin forgiving myself and others. Once I was willing to let go of the negative energy behind all the stories, attitudes and beliefs, miracles lined up for me. It continues to amaze me how well this works. I've changed a lot. I'm happier and healthier now. I exercise a half hour in the morning and dance for a half hour in the afternoon.

I've come to realize that if you want to stay fat forever the most effective thing you can do to maintain and increase those extra pounds is to constantly criticize yourself and your body. The bathroom scales are a wonderful tool to help you along with that. I'm speaking here from years of experience. And as someone once said "If you continue to do what you've always done, you'll continue to get what you've always gotten".

Diets

I see people in the news that have dropped a bundle of weight in what seems like no time. I realize impatience is the American way when it comes to dieting, and that was me in the past. The weight loss never lasted for any length of time though. I'd barely wave hello at the low number on the scales and then I'd start gaining the pounds back. And of course you gain it back. It's logical because diets are no fun. The main premise is to deny yourself the enjoyment of eating. That's not for me ever again. I'll just keep going happily on my way. I'm feeling good, enjoying my food and trusting the extra weight will come off in its own good time.

I'm struck by all the weight loss products on the market today. All promise one thing, speed, and in most cases that is an accurate statement. The only trouble is you'll gain those lost pounds right back again, feel more depressed and have to go searching for another wonder diet you can lose weight on in a matter of weeks. No wonder we keep hearing diets don't work. A lifestyle change is the only true way to do it, especially if you have been chronically overweight like me.

The good news with a lifestyle change is you'll never have to endure another crazy diet. The way I'm eating now is very enjoyable, and if I don't really like what I'm eating I throw it out. I know the weight will never come back because I see no reason to ever change the way I do food again. It is truly one of life's great pleasures. And more and more I am convinced that dropping the guilt and negativity I was so tightly wrapped in is the key. Loving yourself is so important and vital to success.

Here's something I'd like to recommend. Go to the bathroom mirror, look into your eyes and give yourself a standing ovation. Clap . . . clap loud. You deserve it. It brings happy tears to my eyes every time I do it.

The Generator

Sometimes I play solitaire on my p.c. The game is okay but the main reason I play is to check on my subconscious. When I'm relaxed and playing the game all sorts of thoughts drift through my mind. In the past I could find axes to grind and spend a lot of time doing just that. My mom and dad used to say "Thoughts are things". And I believed that but didn't do much about it. Sometimes a rotten thought would get in my head and it was like a runaway train. Thoughts are things and they generate power. I think it's good to think of ourselves as generators especially when we are in state of relaxed concentration or meditating.

I hear people say how hard it is to change, or in most cases they simply say "I can't". They say their circumstances prohibit them from changing because it would be too difficult or too costly or their family and friends wouldn't like it. I've come to realize that new challenges don't have to be negative along the way. My affirmation that a food lifestyle would come to me in an easy, natural, happy, healthy way came to me exactly like that. As my kids use to say, "It's been cinchy".

Start new endeavors with an affirmation that all will come together perfectly using your own words. Your words have powerful energy. Use and feel those affirmations, particularly when you're worried or scared about something. Plant stars around your dreams or concerns by using words like successful, safe, smooth, totally doable and support is all around me.

Positive thinking doesn't work well if, in your gut, you don't think you are worthy or you are in the habit of playing victim. You have to change those beliefs about yourself. You have your very own generator. Use it wisely.

One day I received spam (junk mail) that said "Never be powerless again. Buy a generator." That brought a big smile to my face. I've got one that's built in and it's free. Such a deal!

I saw a demonstration of a generator working while playing cards with my son Dave. The object of the game was to hold a count of 31 in your hand. Along with that you could get three of kind and you'd have 30 and were pretty much assured of winning the hand. But that was a much more difficult and a long shot with only one deck. Well he kept repeating he wanted three of a kind. Not going to happen I thought. He kept repeating it over and over and we tried to convince him that wasn't going to happen. Well after a couple hands he turns up with three of a kind and won. Everyone but Dave was really surprised. But what really came as a shock was he won the next two hands the same way, three of a kind.

I'm not advocating that you do this at Vegas because there are probably a lot of other people at the tables that are doing the same thing. But it can't hurt either. The vast majority of us go through life semi-conscious.

So we need to make the conscious choice to eliminate negative thinking in our lives. For sure we never want to criticize our body or anyone else's again. We are human and slip up sometimes but be aware of how you're feeling when you do that. It doesn't feel good. It gets easier after awhile to stay positive and inevitably life changes.

I watched a TV program called Nova one night and a scientist said that our bodies contain atoms that have particles of energy and these particles use this energy to communicate with other particles to get the innumerable jobs done in our bodies to keep us alive. They are also sending energy outside the body. Wow! So it follows that our thoughts count all the time.

The thing I find interesting about that is why doesn't positive energy work all the time. It could be our lifestyle doesn't jive with our desires and dreams or our core belief isn't in harmony with our wishes. Maybe we're just too scared or unconscious to get it right. Believe me, I understand. Its pretty impossible to think positive thoughts when an elephant is standing on your foot.

I think that's why meditation, prayers, affirmations and gratitude in our daily lives are so important. Those things sustain us when the going gets rough.

What happens when we send prayers to someone else? It appears some people absorb that positive energy and others don't. The truth is it's none of our business once we do our transmitting. We need to accept that. Everyone has their own path to follow and sometimes it doesn't include our wishes.

We've all heard about people that have beat the odds, especially in regards to health issues. I don't think doctors have ever disputed that attitude has a lot to do with that. And what is attitude? It's a consistent way of thinking, and not just when you're sick but while cleaning up the kitchen or waiting in line at the store. The generator is always working.

Bob The Bathroom Scales

What a crazy relationship I have had with Bob over the past months. It has been very much like being in love with a man. At first I couldn't believe I was so lucky as weight began melting away. But then there were the ups and downs of our relationship. One day I'd think: I love you, love you, love you.!!! Another day it would be: Get away from me NOW!!!

I remember a few times I actually banged my head against the wall after an encounter with Bob. During the downs Bob often stayed in his man cave (also more commonly known as the cabinet with the toilet bowl cleaner in it) while I gave him the silent treatment.

When the numbers made me happy I kept Bob out where I could love and enjoy him. Other times he spent considerable time in his cave while I felt (a) bitterly disappointed, (b) cheated (c) totally mystified or (d) just plain pissed off. Does this sound familiar to anyone else?

I can find the humor in it now. And I also see something else. What was I thinking? Well, most of the time it was negative energy. I already knew negatives never help anything and certainly not weight loss. And does Bob actually have the ability to give a flying fig how I feel? I don't think so.

The Cheese Family

Before I go any further I'll introduce you to a family I've had in my head for several years. They are a family of mice and represent wisdom and humor and also the past to me. They will turn up occasionally with comments.

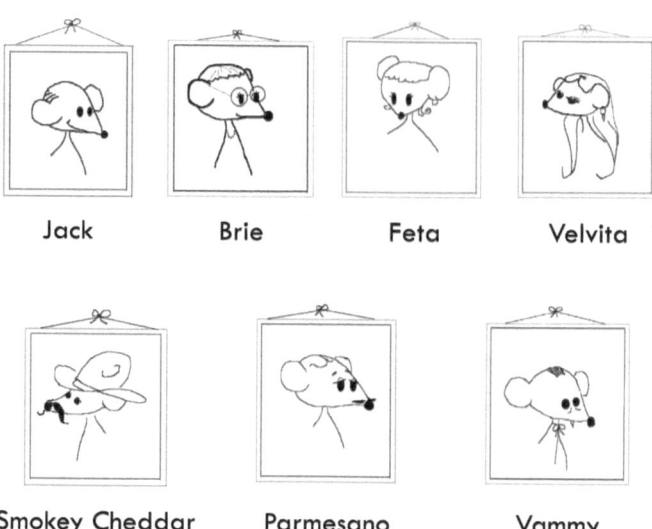

Jack   Brie   Feta   Velvita

Smokey Cheddar   Parmesano   Vammy

Jack Cheese: Jack owns a Thoughts R Us store. He has a good grasp of inventory but still has some beliefs in layaway.

Brie Cheese: Jack's wife. Brie manages the layaway department at Thoughts R Us. It's a big job.

Tillamook Cheese: Tilly is Jack and Brie's daughter, the wife of **String Cheese** and mother of four year old twins **Colby** (Cole) and **Camembert** (Cam) and eight year old **Fondue**.

Velvita Cheese: Jack and Brie's younger daughter. She has a big role on one of the soaps on TV and worries incessantly about her weight.

Smokey Cheddar: Smokey is from Lubbock, TX and is Jack's uncle. He writes songs for the Nashville Sound occasionally.

Parmesano: Parmy is Velvita's long suffering love interest. He is an opera star that has been in many tragic operas.

Vammy: Vammy is a vampire mouse and Jack's distant cousin. He has chronic indigestion.

PART II

The Journal

A new day

Yesterday wasn't my best day living with this new lifestyle. I ate more than I really wanted and I didn't control my thoughts in the afternoon. Today will be better, probably even a really great day.

A new day

I found myself having some critical and judgmental thoughts in the last days. I see people on the news and elsewhere that aren't playing by the rules. How easy it is to get up on my high horse. Yet I have cheated in times without number with my diets. I have to admit it's the same thing only on a smaller scale. Do I forgive those people and dump criticism? I don't think I need to excuse what they are doing but I do need to let go of any negative energy on it. That isn't part of my path.

A new day

I need to work on overeating, especially at the evening meal. Even though it was just roasted vegetables, I ate more than I needed. I don't know where that came from. There was always plenty of food around when I was growing up. My dad was the manager of a Safeway store. I think I was walling off my feelings with food and fat.

A new day

I listened to my body at dinner last night. I noticed that I don't have to eat as much and I like that. My favorite affirmation: Life is good and it just keeps getting better and better.

A new day

Have to stay conscious. More than 70 years of eating when I'm not hungry is my biggest challenge right now. The only reason I eat breakfast is to quiet the hunger pangs, and by lunch I don't seem to have a problem staying on track. Dinner is when I need to improve my awareness. I'm enjoying drinking hot lemonade after dinner. It satisfies my sweet tooth and I read somewhere that lemons deter cancerous growths. So now I drink hot lemonade instead of coffee.

A new day

Sometimes I think it must be nice to be one of the Canadian geese that fly over Durango. I've heard that they are quite democratic and all that honking is about casting their vote on which way to fly and who is up to buck the headwinds and lead the flock. They have more than instinct and democracy going on too. They also have a steady awareness of landmarks on those long flights.

I'm more aware these days but my head still has to catch up with me sometimes. Am I thinking negative? Am I eating more than I need? Or am I letting my mind wonder again? I'll bet a couple of those geese at the end of the vee formation let their little minds wonder sometimes too.

A new day

I am surprised how well staying conscious works. That sounds like a redundant statement but it's true.

A new day

I continue to be conscious of my body when eating. I'm always reminding myself I don't have to eat anything I don't really want and it's liberating. I'm surprised my old issues have dropped by the wayside so easily. This is the most enjoyable diet I've ever been on. And I notice when my mind zeros in on negatives. Easier to spot and reject now.

A new day

When I was in school my friends and I nurtured sarcastic humor. I see that being critical and sarcastic is something I want to stay away from whether it's aimed at myself or anyone else. That needs monitoring, especially when I'm watching TV. In the past it was something of a sport to watch TV and sit and criticize or feel superior to others.

A new day

Stay aware. Wow, that is a loaded one for me. Constantly doing that now and I'm glad. I was thinking this morning about eating fast. I'm always having to remind myself to slow down.

A new day

Still eating whatever I want but I notice I spend a lot more on produce and fish than I did before. I was wondering yesterday if the day would come when I just wanted to rebel and eat anything I wanted. But I'm eating as much of whatever I want now so what is there to rebel about? And there's another plus, I feel better after eating. No more antacids.

A new day

I noticed I didn't like generic shredded wheat at breakfast today. Tasteless. I think I'm getting picky and that's a good thing. In the past I just ate everything in front of me and ignored thoughts if I noticed I didn't really like it or my body was telling me I was full. What a change. I'm continuing to remind myself to stay conscious and aware when eating and it's working.

A new day

I continue to be surprised at how little my stomach needs to be happy. The refrigerator and pantry door swung open pretty often in the past. Anyway last night I had a shrimp cocktail and half a bagel and it held me nicely till this morning. Life is good and it just keeps getting better and better. And being conscious is getting easier. I hear my head telling me that I don't need to hurry eating even if I'm really hungry. There is plenty of time. I also hear myself asking if I really want that bite. Maybe not. You know what? I think I'm wearing a new head and I like it. I guess I'm losing weight there too.

A new day

I'm finding I need to adjust my grocery shopping. Today I bought a container of dehydrated vegetables to take the place of tortilla chips. Don't care for the flavor. They tasted like chemicals to me and I threw them out. I'm still hungry for fish but the frozen fish that comes breaded is not what I want either. And living in Colorado I don't expect fresh fish at the market.

I don't know where they find those tiny pieces of fish that make a sardine look huge in the frozen fish packages. I might as well just fry up some bread crumbs for dinner and be done with it.

A new day

I bought generic shredded wheat cereal last week. May as well have just bought the box and chewed on that. The cereal was devoid of flavor. Along with nonfat milk it's just no fun to eat. I like to enjoy eating now so I mixed granola with raisins and added it to the tasteless stuff. Still hate wasting food. I'm learning.

A new day

Today I poured myself what I thought was a medium bowl of cereal. By the time I was half done my stomach said that was enough. I've sent a fair amount of food down the garbage disposal lately but better it than me. The only time I don't find this easy is when I'm starved at dinner time or when I'm dining with someone. That's when my ability to stay conscious when eating is at its lowest. Reminds me of my grandsons when they were babies. They waved their arms and kicked their legs when food came into view. They got so excited. I don't do that anymore but I do need to settle down and stay conscious.

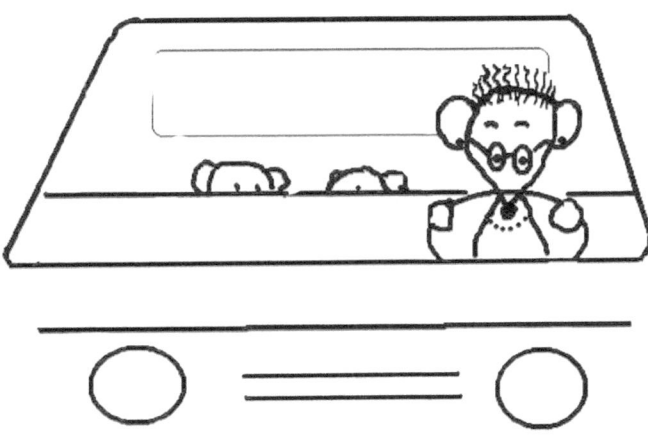

Brie: Okay boys. Quiet down back there so I can drive. Think some happy thoughts.

Cole: No problem grandma. Soft voices coming from the back seat:

Cam: Cole?

Cole: What?

Cam: Hold still so I can eat your arm.

Cole: Grandmaaa!!!!

There's nothing like a couple of little kids to make you stay conscious.

A new day

I ate more than I needed again last night. I will overcome this old habit. No problems the rest of the time. I find what works for me is eating small amounts about four times a day. I'm still learning.

A new day

No problem with dinner last night. I had a shrimp cocktail and green salad. Hot lemonade for dessert. Just right.

The problem that did show up today was when I was in a conversation with friends and some negative thoughts came out of my mouth. I realize I have to be conscious of the thoughts that comes out. I am amazed at how semi conscious I've been much all my life. Sigh.

A new day

Everything is going along great. My stomach is growling this morning. I think I'll have an egg with some hash browns and toast. Yum.

A new day

Was thinking this morning that for the first time in my 75 years I'm eating the way I want to. I'm picky now. I find the courage to throw out or give away food I don't like or don't want. I am enjoying eating. A part of that is staying conscious. I love not eating more than I need or something I don't particularly like. I can remember thinking in the past that sometimes eating seemed kind of like a job.

A new day

I've had a manual treadmill for a couple weeks now. I knew I needed exercise. I'd like to be outside walking. But here in Durango in the winter there is often snow on the ground and being from Southern California I worry about slipping and falling on the ice. And in the warmer weather the bears like to take a stroll too. The locals don't worry about them. I'm just a cautious newcomer.

I have the treadmill now. However it's set on a permanent incline which has me huffing and puffing in no time. I guess these lungs spent too much of their life at sea level. It's about 6,500 feet here in Durango. Excuse? Maybe. I'm timing myself on the thing now and figure that will help me to stretch my abilities. I did it this morning and am embarrassed to say I only lasted three minutes. I'll try for four minutes tomorrow.

A new day

I continue to get pickier about food. I keep trying prepared frozen fish and have either given it away or dumped it. Don't like it or it's too breaded. I'm so hungry for fish but where do you find good ocean fish in Colorado? I guess I'll stick to canned albacore and frozen shrimp.

Made it to five minutes on treadmill today. Puff puff. I'll improve.

A new day

It's all getting easier. Been over a month since I started this new life and I find it pretty easy to discard negative thoughts before they spend any time with me. I like what Deepak Chopra says about negative thoughts. He says we all have them but when they turn up all we have to say is "Next?". I use to be pretty critical or sarcastic about people I connect with or who were on TV. Now I catch it fast and discard it.

The great thing about this "diet" is I can eat as much of anything I need or want. I have really enjoyed my meals. I find I'm fixing yummy and healthy things for myself. Still shocked at how little of it I want or need. And at dinner I need to remind myself it's okay to throw out food. Now though I take smaller portions so waste isn't that much of an issue.

A new day

Up to six minutes on the treadmill. My legs are twitching. It's going to be a few weeks (okay, months) before I make it to 30 minutes. That's okay. I'm in no hurry.

Stomach is starting to growl. Think I'll have the only breakfast I like today, half a bagel, egg and hash browns. Thinking this morning how much I've cut back on flour and sugar products. I still like them but they don't seem to call to me like before.

A new day

Up to eight minutes on treadmill. Are we having fun yet? So far exercise hasn't come as natural as my change in attitudes about diet. Wonder what I can do about that. I'll take it under advisement.

All else is going swimmingly although I did have a thing happen the other day that really got under my skin. I thought a good friend was ignoring me and it hurt my feelings. After journaling about it I realized hurt feelings are ego raising its ugly head. I know that ego is never my friend. Once I got that I felt a lot better. Later I talked to my friend and found that ignoring me wasn't her intention at all and we are fine again

A new day

Is ego ever a good thing to have going on? I can't think when. I know when I've done my best efforts it hasn't been out of ego but out of love. I remember how obsessive I was about perfection when painting a portrait. But my ego was always parked in Cincinnati and love was the dominant factor. I've always defined bliss in those terms, park your ego out of town and give the experience your all.

A new day

The conversations I'm having in my head have sure changed. Today when deciding whether to eat an elderly banana or not I heard: "You don't have to eat that. If you don't want it, throw it out". I did.

A new day

One of the reasons I like the way this "diet" is I can go out to lunch with friends and order whatever I want. Today a friend is making lunch for a group of us. I'm looking forward to it.

Are other women like me? I wouldn't think of overeating when I'm with friends or family. Women just don't do that when there are witnesses. We wait till we're alone to eat crazy. That was me.

A new day

Yesterday I decided to go to Subway for lunch. The spicy Italian is my favorite. I ordered the foot long. I have a strategy. I eat half of it after tearing off the top part of the bun. Too much bread for my taste. And I save the filling for dinner or lunch the next day. It makes a delicious antipasto salad. Two meals. Not bad and suits me just fine.

A new day

I had a dream last night about a friend. She looked like she had lost a lot of weight from the front but her back end was still the same. I laid in bed wondering what to think about that. I suspect that person was me and I still had something in my past that needed attention. Maybe that sounds farfetched but whether it applies to the dream or not there is some truth in the assumption.

I do have a couple of issues that need to be consciously discarded. One of them is the treadmill and exercise. I don't remember ever having a positive thought about exercise. It was all negative. I am changing my attitude about that. No more negatives, thank you very much. I don't have to enjoy it but I need to appreciate it.

A new day

Went to Canyonlands National Park with family. What spectacular scenery and fun to be with them. No problems with thoughts or food. I continue to enjoy eating only what I like or feel the body needs. I remember when I had to eat what I didn't like and ate everything in sight. No more.

I began having some thoughts this morning that were on the critical side. Not about the family but others. People often fall into the criticism habit. It's so easy. I managed to dismiss those thoughts and reminded myself that it's none of my business.

A new day

All my life I've found that when I'm really tired I want to inhale carbs. Sometimes I'd eat them all day long. I'm dealing with that today. The only options for breakfast were cereal or half a bagel. Chose the bagel with berry jam. Will see how the day goes.

A new day

Everything went well yesterday. No problem with carbs.

Been thinking a lot about what happened when I did that mirror work. What seems clear to me now is recognizing the guilt I had wrapped around me all my life that I didn't even know was there. Thankfully I was ready to let that go and that's when the authentic me began to emerge, the me that doesn't have to eat a lot of what I don't need or like. It's still pretty shocking. I eat what I want and need and throw away or give away what I don't.

A new day

I'm finding I taste the chemicals in food now and I don't like them. I want real food, preferably organically grown. I am so lucky to live in Durango. It is one of the epicenters of organic farmers and grass-fed beef. I can enjoy fruits and vegetables without wondering what country they came from and how they were processed. I understand it's sometimes unavoidable but thank goodness for locally grown.

A new day

Hungry all afternoon yesterday so I ate a quarter of a cheese and ham quesadilla and some steamed asparagus about 3:00 p.m.. Didn't want much for dinner. Had a small helping of a frozen pasta dinner with vegetables. Didn't really like it and threw out most of it. I'm not going to eat stuff I don't like anymore, especially processed food.

I'm going to break down and buy a scale today. Curiosity is getting the best of me. I don't expect it will effect how I eat now. There is nothing to be disappointed about or over elated about. But inquiring minds want to know.

A new day

I was thinking again this morning about my "diet". I noticed the one thing missing that has never happened. I never deny myself what I want to eat. I don't stay away from any foods. I don't feel bad if I eat something that is high in calories. Desserts, rich food, it doesn't matter. I stay true to what this body wants. As for sweets, one cookie is enough. And a small hamburger patty and small salad does it for dinner. Before that it would translate to a burger with everything on it, fries and a diet coke. Staying conscious while eating is a big key.

My mother was an extremely slow eater. I'd like to be more like her in that respect. Actually, there are a lot of ways I'd like to be more like her. She had an inherent wisdom about life. She was raised in the Pacific Northwest and when she was a girl there were lots of Nez Perce Indians around. One of the traditions the Indians and she imparted to us as kids was to take what you need but leave the place the way you found it. That means a lot to me. There are a lot of people in various industries I wish would be more like the Indians.

A new day

Thinking back on the years past when weight was never far from my mind. I sometimes weighed twice a day, kept food diaries, and listened to "experts" that had never in their life had a weight problem. I envied all the people that had no idea what it was like being overweight. No more.

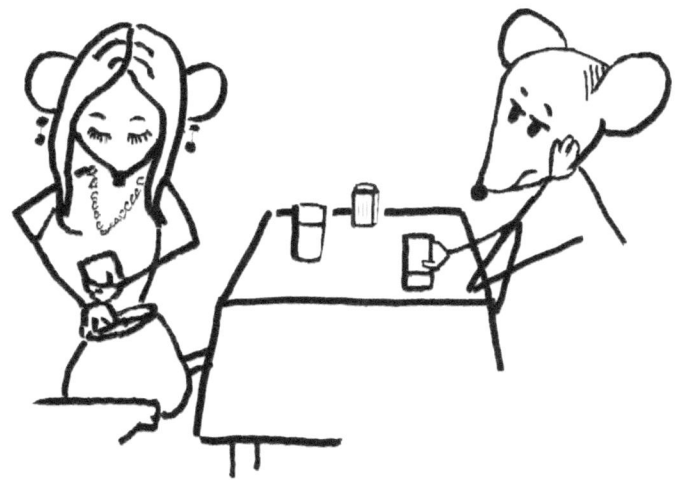

Velvita: Don't go away dad. I want to show you something. It's an anatomically correct chart of all the places I need to lose weight. She hands him the chart. Jack glances at it and starts to hand the chart back.

Velvita: You can keep it. I made 40 copies.

Jack: Sighs. Vel, why is it you can be so successful with your career but always be worrying about your weight.

Velvita: I know. I ought to have Uncle Smokey write a sad song about me. I'll have to write and tell him to do that.

Jack: (sarcastically) And be sure to send him a copy of your chart.

Velvita: I already did.

A new day

I'm still learning about myself. I see where I need to grocery shop now. I seldom hit the middle isles of the grocery store any more except for olives, tomato sauce and inedibles. I go up the hill for grass fed beef and local produce at the ranch market.

A new day

This morning I have a clearer understanding of what forgiveness means. I've known for some time that forgiveness doesn't mean excusing what happened. But, even though we've had some painful experiences, we learn from them. What it means to me now is that I just let go of my energy on it and move on.

Plus I keep hearing in my mind that old bible saying "Judge not lest ye be judged". That is a loaded phrase since the person we judge the harshest is ourselves. Anyway, I now get that those people we feel did us wrong were there to help us learn some lesson. It's hard to see that at the time it's happening, especially when you're a little kid. But at some point in life hopefully it sinks in and we can pull out our Get Out Of Jail Now card and move on.

A new day

Life is good and just keeps getting better and better. I know we all get bonked on the head now and then.

But in the meantime I am happy, fulfilled, contented and hugely grateful.

A new day

Negative thoughts have sort of given up on me. At first it was a constant battle to get them to clear out. Don't hear from them much now. However if there is something I need to clean up in my head I get that message loud and clear. I've also had scary thoughts from time to time that need clearing out. It's weird how at times we terrorize ourselves over something that will never happen. That's one of the places affirmations help. Thoughts are things.

A new day

I'm learning to cook all over again. For the many years I've been by myself I got very lazy in the kitchen. Still don't want to spend hours there but I'm finding out how much I enjoy real food rather than processed stuff.

Takes some time cutting up and chopping but it's worth it. It surprises me that the starches and sugars have lost their hold on me too. I have to admit, that I sure enjoy my hash browns in the morning. And it's nice not to feel like I need to eat a dozen cookies just because they are there. Ah, the authentic me!

A new day

I read somewhere that although a torpedo has a direct target it never goes in a straight line. It is constantly correcting itself to allow for currents, weather, etc.

That's where I am right now, doing a little correcting. I have a feeling I'm still eating more than I need from time to time. Need to stay conscious. If I was into tattoos I'd have Stay Conscious printed on the top of my right hand.

A new day

Thinking back I'm trying to remember the longest I ever stayed on a diet. It ranged from one day to maybe two months for me, never ever longer than that. And sometimes I'd be fairly successful for a time. But continuing to be wrapped in the guilt that I wasn't even aware of and the accompanying negativity, there was no way I was ever going to be permanently successful with weight loss because of the label I'd given to myself of failure. The Get Out Of Jail Now card remained there in my back pocket.

A new day

I went to a big birthday party the other day. I loved table hopping and not caring about the table with all the munchies on it. I did try the punch and didn't like it. Picky, picky and that's okay with me. The people were much more fun to visit with. I have to admit that I didn't first walk out my front door remembering to stay conscious. Happily it was a wonderful day anyway. Next time I'll do better.

A new day

I continue to play like I'm a torpedo. I know where I'm going and I'm aware when I'm drifting off course. And that's good. I'm conscious of it and do a little correcting. Sometimes I doubt myself. Maybe I'm just not doing life right. But then I think about how happy I am and I continue on my merry way.

A new day

Not my finest moment yesterday. An assistant at an office I called discovered my pet peeve which is when they insist on talking even though I try to inject a question or remark. Do they teach that in school these days? If you talk loud enough and fast enough the person on the other end of the conversation must shut up apparently. Why does this rudeness get under my skin so much?

I was brought up to have civil give and take conversations. I started yelling at the assistant and she just kept right on talking only louder. Lord I was disgusted. Finally I just shut up and listened and she just kept on talking. Sigh. How should I have reacted to this? Not by yelling and thinking negative thoughts. Will have to think more on this.

A new day

I thought about my yelling match with the office clerk. I realized my ego was doing the yelling and not my upbringing. When I recognized that, it pretty much deflated all the energy I had spent on that. I didn't need to sign on to her problem.

I will just shed that kind of thing in the future . . . I hope. It's interesting how you keep learning about yourself even well into your years. I'm glad.

A new day

I've taken up crocheting. I feel like the character in Tale of Two Cities, Madame DeFarge. She knit all of the names of the people that were doomed to be beheaded into her quilt during the French Revolution. However, I try to keep my thoughts on a positive note. It's very therapeutic for me. She probably thought so too. Hate has the ability to energize you, but oh what a price we pay later. Negative thoughts are just downright expensive.

A new day

Ten weeks since this all began. It has been so great learning about my authentic self. I like refusing to eat what I don't like or need. And I've never had to beat myself up for eating something like the candy corn I had yesterday. I look at my grocery list and I see a lot of fish and produce now.

I have a bit of a hard time eating beef. I buy the grass fed variety at James Ranch market near where I used to live. The cattle grazed in the pasture in the Animus Valley there by my windows. I've struggled with a vague feeling I'm eating my neighbors. Yuck! But I've managed to get over it mostly. But I suspect I will start living without meat in the future.

Breakfast continues to be a task for me. I just don't like breakfast food except the occasional egg and hash browns. Cereal and sweets don't appeal to me.

A new day

I continue to use the treadmill. Thinking back I realize not once in my life have I had anything positive to say about working out. It's always been something I forced myself to do occasionally. I'm coming out of that attitude now. It's all part of my diet of negative thoughts. So I tell myself I really appreciate the opportunity to exercise and am thankful for the good it does me. Maybe I don't enjoy it but I am grateful.

A new day

After reading through this journal one thing is clear, dinner is the time I most often make mistakes. I often tell myself that just because it tastes good that doesn't mean I have to eat it all. That sounds strange to a normal person but to me it's inherent. I guess I'm a bit compulsive.

I so admire my little grandsons. They listen to their body and obey. When they've had enough to eat they just shake their head no or hold up their hand in refusal. I want to retrieve that kind of wisdom.

A new day

Last night after dinner my mind said I wanted more. And with this diet I told myself I could have anything I wanted or needed if I'd just wait a few minutes and made sure I was still hungry. I did that and then went to the refrigerator for some watermelon. I was happy after that. I love this diet a lot.

A new day

"You don't have to eat all of this even though it tastes especially good to you." That's what I heard in my head this morning as I was eating cheese toast and half an apple. So I left half my breakfast on the plate and I was satisfied. I made too much and now it will go down the garbage disposal. Next time I'll make less. What a concept, staying conscious when eating.

A new day

It's been nearly three months now. I'm glad I bought the scale because it is a delight stepping on Bob every week and seeing the weight drop. And there's never a reason to reprimand myself for something I've chosen to eat.

Food is no longer the enemy. I love that. I've been toying with the idea of making myself some hot chocolate with brandy some evening. Maybe tomorrow.

A new day

I had hot chocolate with brandy last night. Yum. It's even good with nonfat dry milk. I'll have to remember that for next winter.

A new day

Before I did my exercises this morning I thought I was starved. All I thought about was food. But then after I'd finished those things I sat down here at the computer and my first thought was about breakfast and I felt like I could take it or leave it. So now that it's okay with me to eat, I don't care about it. What is up with that?

A new day

Last night I had a bad time of it. I began doubting myself big time. Maybe I'm not doing life right at all I thought.

Are the changes I've made going in the right direction? Maybe I'm just deluding myself. During this and after a few tears my head kept telling me not to entertain such thoughts. They were taking me in the wrong direction and are costly. I finally gave it up and went to bed.

I know I really need to keep my mind on mindless games and fluff TV that time of night. My mind energy level just isn't as strong then as during the day and early evening.

My grandsons have had sweet stories read to them every night at bedtime since they were about four or five months old. What a good idea that is. Do they write sweet bedtime stories for adults?

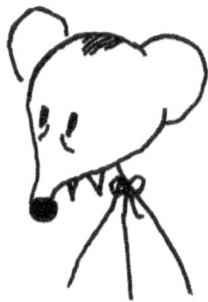

I hope so. I'm getting sick and tired of your blood type.

A new day

After nearly three months of living in this new head of mine I see there are two things that need to happen in order to shed weight and keep it off.

The first thing is to face yourself head on (in my case it was in front of the bathroom mirror) and acknowledge what's stopping you: criticism, resentment, fear or guilt. I'm betting in most cases it's guilt that we took on as little kids and never recognized. Then we must be willing right then and there to let go of it and forgive ourselves. And you are not the guilty party anyway.

The second thing that has to happen is you need to stay conscious when you are eating and keep thinking positive. Listen to the voice in your head that says, "I've had enough or I don't have to eat that if I don't want to or slow down, there is plenty of time or just because it tastes good doesn't mean I have to eat everything in sight".

A new day

I think most people, especially Americans, eat way too fast. The other day I had a McBreakfast and saved the sausage patty for the family dog. He scarfed it down in three seconds flat and I wondered if he had any sensation of what he had eaten. Maybe a second of it in his nose.

I've eaten that way in the past and sometimes I didn't even remember eating. Like my daughter says, we need to be more like the Europeans and really enjoy our food.

A new day

Last night for dinner everything tasted so good. My first impulse was to go for a second helping. Happily my head said no problem. "Eat as much as you want. Just make sure it's because you're still hungry". I realized I wasn't hungry anymore and felt fine about laying my fork down.

A new day

Ahhh. Life is good and it just keeps getting better and better. My family was here for dinner last night. It was good to have them all here with me. My eight year old grandson played a great game of baseball before dinner but the game wasn't over until 7:00 p.m. I got to see what happens when I am tired and starved. I wolfed down practically everything on my plate.

I was about 90% unconscious of what I was consuming. Thankfully I didn't eat the chips or dessert. I'll do better when conditions like that come up again.

A new day

I went out for dinner last night. I was more conscious this time and didn't eat everything in sight. I enjoyed a few nacho chips and didn't feel guilty about it. Restaurants serve such huge portions these days. No wonder so many of us are overweight.

A new day

Oh boy. This afternoon I ate half a banana, or at least I think I did. It was in my hand and then I looked down and it was gone. Drat. I had gone unconscious again. I'll do better tonight. I continue to enjoy eating these days, especially when I stay conscious. I fix simple meals but they taste so good. I know what I want now. Mostly fish and produce although I enjoy beef now too. I think I'll start making open faced sandwiches, maybe egg or tuna or lettuce and tomatoes in the mornings. The breakfast police can think what they want, I just don't care. This is the easiest and hardest diet I've ever lived with. Ah well, time for a nice glass of wine.

A new day

Beautiful day. Decided to make hamburger patties and stew them in mushrooms cooked in butter, garlic and white wine and have some home make coleslaw for dinner. Yum. Yes, I plan my meals ahead of time because I want something I'll truly enjoy rather than just grabbing something out of the fridge. I was going to make my own salad dressing with white wine but bought some of Paul Newman's dressing instead. I like that all profits from that company go to charity.

A new day

I think the food editor in my head is getting louder. Or maybe I'm just listening closer. So often I hear "Are you sure you're still hungry? Eat only if you feel you need it". What an important key that is. I never ever deny myself food if I feel hungry. And also there is no reason to be greedy.

A new day

I woke up late today and never got hungry till afternoon. I had lunch about 1:00. The breakfast police must hate me. Tough toenails.

Yesterday I bought one of those little watermelons that are the size of a cantaloupe. It was sweet and juicy, but the heart of it was mealy and the color was off. Made me wonder if it was a one of those things they were tinkering around with in some lab.

That's another reason to refuse to eat certain foods. I just don't feel right about it and down it went into the garbage disposal. If I'm going to eat one I want it to be real not something out of a laboratory.

I suppose those kinds of things have their place but not on my plate. So now the reasons I refuse food are: I don't like it, I don't need it or I just don't feel right about it.

A new day

It's so important to stay away from negative thinking. It's easy to say, not always so easy to do.

I've been annoyed a couple times in the last weeks and find myself up on my high horse. I've brushed it off but it took some conscious effort. I know negative thinking is an expensive luxury I don't want to pay for.

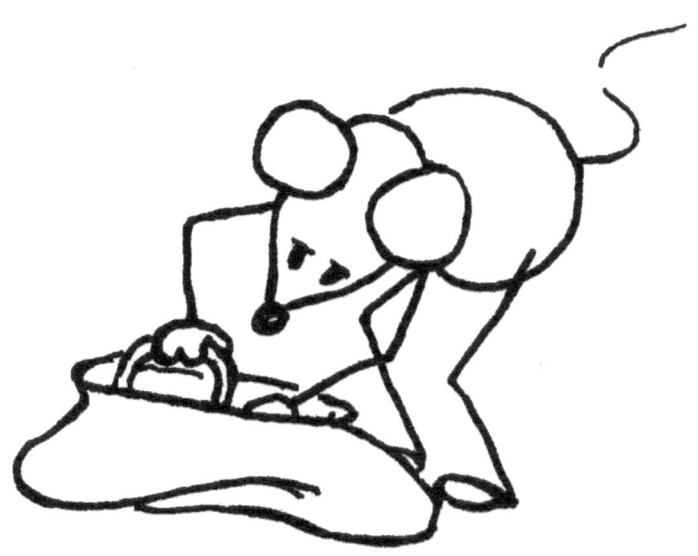

Fondue: What all's in that big ole bag granddad?

Jack: Oh, my cowboy boots, diamond encrusted cheese cutter, golf cl . . . .

Fondue: Granddad!! Nobody owns a diamond encrusted cheese cutter, especially not a mouse!

Jack: rummages through his bag. Alright!! I wondered where my skis were. Ah, here it is. He holds up the cheese cutter.

Fondue: No fair granddad. That is so wrong. I don't even have enough money to buy a brownie. What are you pinning on my shirt? I feel like I'm being deputized.

Jack: You are. It's a badge that says "The Law Acts On My Word."

A new day

Ouch. I thought I was doing the right thing. Even checked with someone else who agreed it was the right thing to do. Turns out it was definitely the wrong thing to do. Now I don't know what I should have done, if anything. Later someone offered me a cookie. I think I ate it because it's gone. Rats. Rats. Rats. Ah well, tomorrow will be better.

A new day

The thing I've learned from yesterday's experience is that everyone has a right to their opinion and I'm not the only one who has painful issues to deal with.

My head has been telling me something new the last couple days while eating. Experience your food. Who does that? Americans sure don't. Nearly all of us choke down our food, especially if it's a familiar food and we already know we like it. I gave it a try at lunch time today. Found out the bread was almost tasteless but was okay with the egg salad. I'll skip it next time though and make croutons out of the bread instead. At least I can enjoy the crunch. I'm glad to be away from diet pop and all its chemicals.

Speaking of chemicals I went to the store for tortillas the other day. Spent ten minutes going through all the brands trying to find one that didn't have an inch and a half of ingredients listed. Why do they put all those chemicals in a simple tortilla? Thankfully the health food stores carry real tortillas with only three or so ingredients. I appreciate that.

A new day

Yuk! I was foolish enough to buy generic cheerios. They sucked up the milk and got mealy before I even had a chance to taste them. I gave the rest of the box away.

When will I learn about generic stuff? And don't those food producers have test kitchens? Stewed some raspberries and added a little sugar. The cereal and berries were so tasty this morning with walnuts and wheat germ. I'll do that again.

A new day

I've been thinking again about negative thoughts and how if we send them out they come back and bonk us on the nose. I see them now as expensive thoughts. Am I willing to pay the price for them? Of course not.

A new day

I recognize negative thoughts pretty fast now. When something unpleasant or odd happens to me now I know I need to identify what I've been thinking. The one thing I notice getting in my way from time to time is my ego. That gets me into mischief sometimes, and I need to stay conscious about that one.

A new day

I met with Bob this morning and found I'd gained a pound this week. I didn't do anything different so I'll just trust my body and trust it knows what it's doing. I won't change anything since I remain content with the way I'm eating. Nothing much has changed for weeks. I have very light meals at night. I often just have a green salad or soup. The rest of the day is the usual. I think my favorite thing for lunch these days is egg salad.

A new day

I continue to eat whatever I want. It was my birthday this week. Don't care much for cake so Heidi made a peach pie. It was delicious but not in the way it was in the past. I could pretty much take it or leave.

The weight loss continues slowly but so what. I know I'll get where I want to be. And after that I'll continue eating this way for the rest of my life because I'm happy and enjoying it.

A new day

Yesterday I spent time with some really nice people. But the conversation got pretty negative and I went unconscious and joined in. I don't want to do that again. It's easy when I'm alone to stay on track. I know right away now when I'm off track. I lose my happy.

Lately I've experienced some worry about family. Mothers are like that. Worry is another form of negative thought though and I need to pay more attention to the warning flag in my mind. Better to just do some affirmations and send a load of love when that shows up again.

As for falling into line with someone else's negative thinking, I'll just keep my mouth shut or change the subject when it happens. Best to be proactive than reactive. I'll do better next time.

A new day

It occurred to me this morning that the comments in my head when I'm eating have quieted down. I have an uneasy feeling that maybe I've been ignoring them. I know that can happen. If you just keep turning off the warnings in your head and go unconscious, after awhile they just stop. Maybe that's how serious addictions start. I have to stay aware. I'll do better today.

A new day

I've decided to aim for two pounds a week with Bob instead of one. The other day a neighbor said she only ate salad or soup for dinner. I think that's a good idea. I'm sure that can hold me comfortably to the next day. If it doesn't I'll eat more (one of the shining points of this diet). The main thing is to lose weight in an easy, natural, happy, healthy way just like I've been doing for the past four months.

A new day

I've been watching chefs judging other chefs on television shows. The food doesn't interest me so much since I won't be putting caramels and clam sauce together any time soon. What interests me are the judge's comments especially when they talk about different textures, layers of flavors and how the plate looks. Ah, to have such an educated palate. Can they really taste all those flavors and notice textures in their mouth? They must take very slow and thoughtful bites. Talk about being conscious. I admire that a lot.

A new day

It's been four months on this "diet" and I celebrated by giving myself a standing ovation in the mirror. I highly recommend everyone do that from time to time. It brought a tear to my eye and made me very happy.

A new day

I keep thinking about our mind as generators. I love that idea because it gives me my authentic power to be proactive rather than reactive with my life. Great minds say we are co-creators of our lives with the universe. What a beautiful concept that is.

A new day

A neighbor gave me two homemade brownies today. I ate one and it was really delicious. She is a great baker. The other one is in the freezer. My favorite sweets these days are fresh Colorado peaches from the produce stand.

A new day

Attended a potluck get-together the other night. Without checking the ingredients on the label I bought some cream cheese to put on celery. It was tasty but when I got home and studied the label I found it was crammed with preservatives and chemicals I couldn't pronounce. I threw out the rest of it. No more of that stuff for me.

A new day

Well drat. I've had shoulder problems for the past few months and at this point I'm unable to use the treadmill.

A new day

Yes! A pound came off today and I'm happy with Bob. I watched a program about dieting today. I am so thankful I don't subscribe to those old ways of thinking any more. People use the word cheating when they don't follow their diet exactly. That makes me cringe because berating yourself never helps. I had no unhappy feelings while eating a brownie yesterday. It tasted great and I have no desire for any more.

A few days ago a friend mentioned she was counting calories, and another friend said she was cutting way back on sugar. For me, criticizing myself and denying myself beautiful food is not the way for me. If I'm hungry I'm going to eat it, enjoy it and bless it to my body. No guilt involved. Oh happy day.

A new day

Ahhh. I had half a pita with a whole tomato and mayo along with some lemonade for breakfast today. Yum. Go fish you breakfast police. I love not having to count carbs, calories or fat grams.

A new day

I continue my mental housecleaning where it concerns thoughts and actions. The other day I discovered a little corner of my mind that I didn't know was still there. That morning there were two parking spaces at the strip mall right together. I let a little sports car coming from the other direction pull in first. He was in a hurry and managed to take two spaces with that little car. Remember that old song of Elton John's, *The Bitch Is Back*? Well . . . I was. I made a sarcastic request for him to move the car into just one space and he did. The truth is I could have made the same request with a friendlier delivery and have had the same results. Rats. Oh well, I'll do better next time.

A new day

In the past I used chocolate chip cookies to medicate myself or something else with chocolate, sugar or white flour in it. I don't think I've used food for anything in these past five months except to enjoy while satisfying hunger. I no longer use it to drown out experiences I don't like. Ah, life is good and it just keeps getting better and better.

A new day

I've about decided to stop setting goals for my weight loss. Bob bounces around so much it's getting frustrating. I think I'll just trust my body to do what it does best, take care of itself. I haven't changed my eating patterns so I don't feel I'm doing anything wrong there.

Sometimes I think about my body and how it is literally made from the stars. How divine is that!

A new day

I was in the weeds last night and early this morning. The family cancelled dinner which didn't set too well since I'd already spent a bundle at the grocery store for special ingredients and the main dish was already made for five people. In truth it was just as well. The flavor didn't suit me at all and I would not have been happy about serving it.

But then a problem arose when I almost fell into my old habit of not wanting to throw it all away. In the past I'd sit down and eat half of it by myself, even though it didn't taste very good. Thankfully everything went down the garbage disposal this time.

Also I started feeling annoyed at the family, me and the dinner I had thrown away. Then this morning it came to me that those were expensive thoughts and I didn't want to pay for them. My attitude changed and I'm happy again.

A new day

My weight loss is acting strange. It's not like past diets. In the past when I was really dieting I'd lose a couple pounds a week. But now I see lower numbers only once or twice a month. The rest of the time it just bounces around. I suspect it has something to do with my age. Oh well, as long as it continues to fall I'm happy. I've decided to throw weight loss goals out the window and just trust my body's wisdom.

A new day

Last night I did something at dinner I've never done before. I stopped eating a small dinner I'd always finished in the past. This time I left about a third of it and I didn't even have to listen to my head. It was just automatic. Maybe I'm catching on to not eating more than I need and the automatic reaction has kicked in. It's good being normal and authentic.

A new day

I got together with Bob today and realized I hadn't weighed in this low for at least eight years. Wow. In the past I would have eased up on the diet with that news. Today I had a fresh peach. Life is good and it just keeps getting better and better.

A new day

I continue to feel amazed at how I eat now. Sugar, white flour and pasta hold no interest for me. I eat them once in a while but it's just not the same. I no longer care about them or other things like fast food, and I am less and less tempted to overeat. I lose weight and still eat whatever I want which is mostly fruits, vegetables and some protein like cheese, nuts, fish and grass fed beef. I like cereal pretty well now that I doll it up. Life is good and it just keeps getting better and better

A new day

Row, row, row your boat gently down the stream.

That's what I was singing to myself at 3:00 a.m. this morning. Couldn't sleep. But something someone said kicked in for me. It was my physical therapist, Jen. (She is helping to get my shoulder healed up for me). One day we were talking about how many years of schooling it took her to get her license as a physical therapist.

I was rather shocked and remarked what a long time that was. She said that was the wrong way of looking at it. She said she knew she was going in the right direction and enjoyed school and the friendships all along the way so the time spent was totally okay with her. It was a part of her life that she said was both fun and difficult.

I thought about that and realized that is exactly the attitude I need to have as I'm in the process of shedding extra weight. My body knows when it's time to let go of a pound or two and I don't need to set any time limits. It is so American to be impatient with this process. We want it all off within weeks like on TV even though it took years to pile on.

And so the message is just keep doing what you're doing because you know you're going the right direction and enjoy yourself along the way. The body in its wisdom will take care of the rest in its own good time.

Thus the song, "Row, Row, Row Your Boat

A new day

Last night I watched a doctor on TV tell how important it is to eat fruits and vegetables and how our health will improve dramatically if we do. I agree. He also mentioned that we eat too much. Again I agreed. The only things he left out were the high cost of negative thinking, how important it is to stay conscious of what's going in our mouth and doing the face off in the mirror. For me those were the dynamite. Without those actions odds are I would be back to the old ways of medicating myself with pasta and chocolate chip cookies.

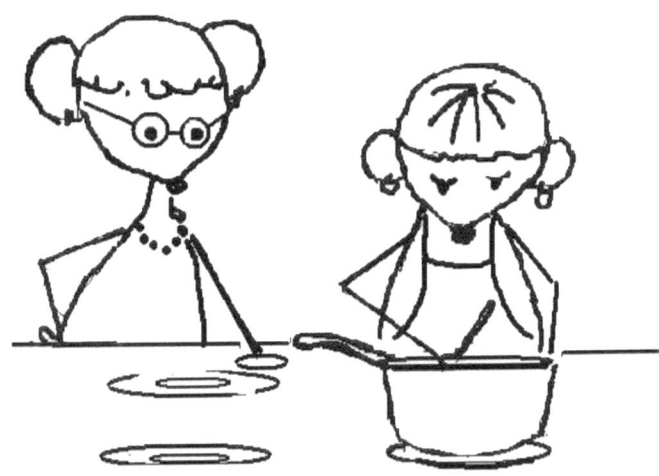

Brie: What's that awful smell Feta?

Feta: It's called Nasty Stew. It's dad's recipe.

Brie: It looks like water. What's in it?

Feta: All my resentments and guilt. It seems like the older they are, the more they smell.

Brie: Well, it's nasty alright. I think you ought to dump the whole thing out and try a new recipe.

Feta: Maybe that's what dad was thinking.

Brie: What?

Feta: He said I'd know it was done when I was ready to dump it.

A new day

The other day I had a thin slice of birthday cake and another day a peach tart. My palate told me I should really like these things but the truth is they left me stuck in neutral. They tasted good but the energy is just gone on pastries for me. I don't dislike them. They are just not important to me anymore. I'm not going to bother with them from now on. I much prefer fresh fruit.

A new day

I like to lay in bed and think things over in the morning before I start the day. Today I gave myself a standing ovation except I was still lying down. It was wonderful. I lay there clapping and smiling to myself. It felt great to feel the love, appreciation and approval of myself. It brought a tear to my eye.

A new day

One of my sweet neighbors offered me some homemade cake today. I thanked her and explained it would be a waste because I just don't have a taste for pastries any more. She appreciated my honesty and found someone else to give it to. I still find it so very strange that that was me saying that. Lord, I used to really be able to put away sugar and flour. I still like sugar in lemonade and stewed with berries, but that's about it. Now my neighbor gives me homemade pickled vegetables. Yum!

A new day

This was a red letter day. All my pants are way too big. They are too long and just draped around me. I took them to the Goodwill and then shopped for new ones.

The new ones will last five to six months and I'll need to discard them and buy a smaller size again. That's fine with me. Who doesn't want to lose weight in their beam. Men I guess. Do they ever use a rear view mirror? Probably only when they look to see if a cop is following them.

Another neighbor came and offered me some peach cobbler today, probably my very favorite dessert in the past.

Since I still have no appetite for pastries I told her it would be wasted on me. She seemed to be okay with that, although she didn't understand it.

I'm getting used to telling people it would be a waste. It is nice of them to offer though.

A new day

I'm getting wise to the ways of my body. This morning Bob said I'd gained three pounds. That's happened before. It reminded me of a story about Chuck Yeager, the first man to break the sound barrier. A reporter asked him what that was like. Yeager said that it was real smooth up there until he hit the barrier and then the plane vibrated like crazy until he had gone through it.

I think life is often like that. The same thing happens with my little grandsons. They are happy little guys until they go through a very grouchy faze just before they make a learning breakthrough. Same with weight loss only with me it's tears. The more weepy I get, the better my life is afterwards.

A new day

I've been reading a book by Eckhart Tolle called *A New Earth*. I've been suspicious of the ego for some time, and now my thoughts are confirmed. Occasionally in the past I felt that one person or another had a big ego. We all have one to deal with and it's a pain in the neck. The times I still beat myself up about something my ego has invariably been involved. It lurks in so many corners of my mind and never serves my best interests. I heard someone say several years ago "Your ego won't be happy with you until you're dead".

With that I'm off to make myself an open faced avocado sandwich with garlic salt and a side of cherry tomatoes. Mmm. One of my favorite lunches.

A new day

Six months now and I'm noticing it's no longer an effort to quit eating when my stomach is satisfied.

I must still need to get used to serving myself smaller portions because quite a bit goes down the garbage disposal. But, I'm sure happy I no longer feel compelled to eat everything in sight.

I've also come to the conclusion that Bob is really unnecessary. Maybe I'll just break up with him. My weight bounces around but I continue losing at a steady pace and my clothes keep getting bigger. I think I'm learning about trust these days.

A new day

I thought I might try out meditation so I've been doing it for the past couple of weeks. My mom and dad practiced it and a lot of other people I respect do it. I may as well be honest, I don't get it. I can come to a very deep state of relaxation just short of sleep, clearing my mind of chatter. But then I sit there and the thought comes to me that this is a very nice place to visit but nobody is home. Why am I here?

So I've decided the answer for me is that I don't need this right now. I'm not saying it's useless for other people but it's just not for me right now.

A new day

Bah. Bob didn't make me happy this morning. I felt discouraged and frustrated. Then I realized that those are negatives and in turn expensive thoughts that I don't want to pay for. Besides I like being happy better than depressed so I changed my thinking.

It occurred to me that I wanted approval from Bob. I've never felt approval was much of an issue for me. When I drew portraits at Knotts Berry Farm my mind was constantly giving me approval, and I didn't need any more from the public. Approval from customers and the onlookers was nice but not that important. However, one day a little four year old girl stood beside me watching silently as I drew her mother's portrait. At length she turned to me and said "That is truly amazin'!!" That remark always bring a big smile to my face.

But Bob is a different story. Bob could very easily make me want to give up when the numbers don't go down like I think they should. How could I give such power to a small appliance? I know I am going in the right direction and I don't need strokes from him. It's fun to see weight loss register but I already knew that. I have learned three things: trust my body, be patient and enjoy the trip along the way. Row, row, row your boat gently down the stream.

A new day

Still singing that song to myself. And I've been thinking this morning about how I reacted to Bob in the past. Mostly I would get disgusted, just give up and begin ignoring him. Also I developed a craving for foods that I had been denying myself. Well, I don't deny myself anything anymore so there are no cravings.

I recognize that my body is quite literally made from the stars and it has an inherent wisdom far beyond my consciousness. It knows what works and lets me know when I was going in the wrong direction.

I'm not ignoring Bob but I am giving him a rest. I think weighing myself once a month is plenty. In fact I don't really need him at all. I'll just go happily on my way buying smaller size pants every once in a while. Life is good and it just keeps getting better and better.

A new day

Sometimes I don't think I'm very good at being human. I acted like a snot head with an Email I sent today. I'll have to clean that up right away.

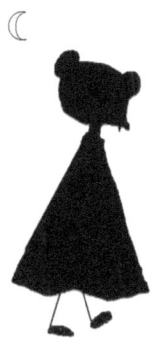

I'm changing my route. Snot doesn't agree with me.

A new day

Taking the energy off Bob's performance is a major change for me. It reminds me of the energy I had on carbs in the past. It's weird how we misplace our sanity.

I find myself thinking of those weight loss programs that demand you exercise five or six hours a day and eat all things dietetic. The universe is masterful at customizing efforts to match each of us so I respect everyone's way of doing things. I'm just glad I'm doing this my way.

Speaking of going your own way, a friend related something to me that I thought was pretty interesting since I like to rub shoulders with folk medicine once in a while. She said her husband had a heart attack and then heard that cayenne pepper was good for the heart. So each morning he filled a capsule with cayenne pepper and took it with water. He lived another forty years without having another heart problem.

I'm no doctor or dietician but it seemed to work for him. It couldn't hurt unless maybe you had a sensitive stomach.

A new day

Been thinking more about attitudes since my ego got kicked in the shins the other day. I've been wondering how to handle that. I'm pretty clear now the ego is never ever my friend. Also thinking a lot about negative thoughts. I've come to realize there are so many ways they show up, criticizing others, thinking the worst is going to happen, living in fear of not having enough of whatever.

Money worries were always one of my favorites. And the more I worried the worse it got. Not being enough was such a constant in my life that I shortened the word to enuf when I was journaling. That one stuck with me for six decades until one day at church the minister said we are all made from the stars. I knew then and there that I was enough and always would be. Not only are we made from the stars but our soul always was, is and will be. Love it.

A new day

My heart is singing for two reasons. One, I will be spending the weekend with the family driving to camp in Moab. It's my grandson's sixth birthday and of course he is all excited. Also, my shoulder is healing and not paining me as much. What a relief that is. Life is good and just keeps getting better and better.

A new day

Yesterday I ate a whole avocado and totally enjoyed it without a minute's worth of remorse. I didn't give a fig how many calories were in it. I love this authentic me and I love the wisdom that is built into my body. I think back how silly it was to be upset when I didn't drop weight when I thought I should have. I trusted my heart to beat every minute of every day. I trusted my bladder to work and my muscles to react when I wanted to move my arm.

What in the world ever made me think I could be smarter than the wisdom of my body and its weight.

I've learned patience since I began this lifestyle. Eat what looks good to me, stay conscious about only eating what I need and my body will take care of the rest. I could give away Bob now because I trust my body. I shed weight when it's time. Yesterday I tried on last winter's coat and it is getting way too big for me. It had been snug around my hips. I'm glad I never got into the habit of arguing with my tape measure. Again, my body has been taking care of business without my nagging.

It all makes me think back a few years ago when I had a stress test. When I was done the technician turned on the computer screen and we watched my heart beating. As I sat there I was filled with awe, love and gratitude. Life is truly a magnificent event.

A new day

Last night I had a hard time quitting eating dinner. I'd made an open faced beef and cheese sandwich and it tasted so good. I wanted to gobble it all down, but then I heard the voice in my head and it was really lecturing me this time. It said "Think of this decision as you would your bank account. Are you making a withdrawal that you can't afford or are you making a deposit that will enhance your currency (trust) in yourself?" And of course, if you are truly still hungry, finish the sandwich. I looked at the leftover half of my dinner and it went down the garbage disposal.

I made a conscious choice to listen to my head while eating months ago and I now realize that when we eat unconsciously like when we eat standing up or in the car, we lose that power of choice and that really goes against my grain. I'm glad I listened.

A new day

How many months has it been now? Seven I guess. What a blessing that "Get Out O f Jail Now" card is. Not only am I losing weight consistently but I've noticed some big lessons along the way. One is trust. I totally trust my body to lose weight in its own good time and it's best to weigh only once a month or so because I've learned that the pounds dance around during the month. I've also learned patience. I know I'm going in the right direction and I'm aware now that there is no hurry. Nature is taking care of business. This is a direct contrast to how I once looked at weight loss; lose it now and lose it fast.

A new day

The autumn leaves outside my windows remind me every day how wise nature is. They also remind me of the old scrub oak that lives where I lived at James Ranch north of Durango. It is the second largest scrub oak in Colorado. It's vast. And it got that way from starting out as a little acorn. Nature took great care of it. It reminded me that when I get impatient or when I want to take control, which is more often than I like to admit, I need to back off.

73

A new day

I've noticed lately that at bedtime I'm just a little bit hungry, and that's okay with me. Once I've brushed my teeth in the evening my mouth is on vacation till the next day. I'm not tempted to go to the refrigerator or pantry. I used to eat pretty much all afternoon though. Now I eat something between 3:00 and 4:00 to hold me till dinnertime. Sometimes a carrot and cheese or an apple and walnuts.

A new day

I often see that I really don't need much at all for dinner in the evening. And it seems curious to me that I can eat a very small meal at night and still not wake up hungry in the morning. In the past I'd sometimes eat a very heavy meal at night and wake up hungry in the morning. It doesn't seem to make sense.

A new day

Nearly eight months now, and I don't know why I'm counting. The body will lose weight in its own good time. I am down two pants sizes now and I am perfectly happy eating this way for the rest of my life.

My heart aches for those who think eating a half of an avocado or a cookie means it's time to beat themselves up. I wish they could understand that food isn't the enemy. That concept is so last century. I eat healthy now and I have never enjoyed food more in my life.

A new day

I've been thinking about chronically overweight people. We have always criticized ourselves and our bodies for being fat. I starved myself, went on countless crazy diets, counted calories, carbs, fat grams and spent money on pills, meetings, mail order food and diet plans only to see a very temporary weight loss. It seemed I was doomed and then went back to hating my body. I think a lot of people feel that way.

A new day

I was talking to the physical therapist about the body yesterday. She is educated in the physiology of the body, and told me about the incredible instrument that the body is, how many functions it must do. The conversation made me remember seeing my own heart beating on the computer screen in real time. It's awe inspiring. It's like our body is a universe there inside and it works day and night with one objective, to keep us alive. How's that for devotion.

It made me think how I have done nothing but criticize my body most of my life. I've often treated it like a piece of trash by eating junk food, processed foods, sweets, way too much pasta, not exercising and then criticize it for not looking the way I wanted it to.

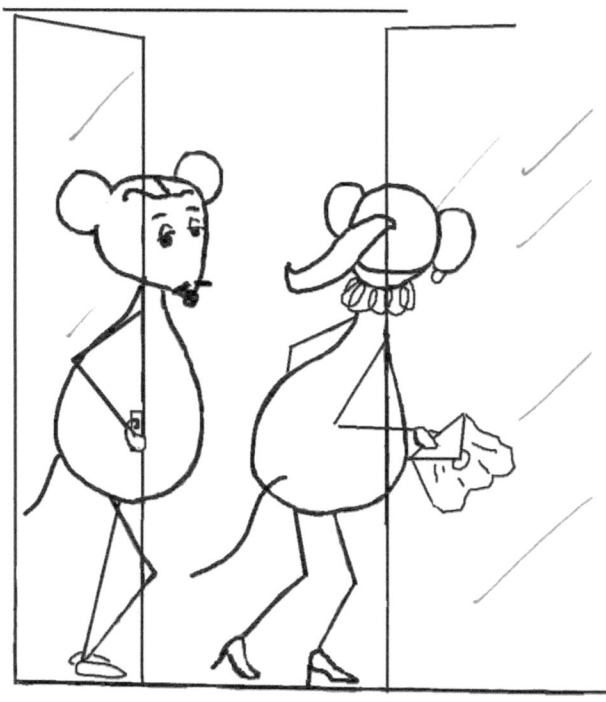

Velvita: Do you think I look fat Parmy?

Parmesano: Of course not cara mia. You are gorgeous, like a perfect pear.

Velvita: WHAT!!!!? Parmy, some people tell me I have the body of Venus!

Parmesano: Of course my darling, just like Venus.

Velvita: Was that so hard? Now open the door for me.

Parmesano: thinks, Still looks like a pear to me.

A new day

Well here's what I'm thinking. How would the body react if we just stopped criticizing it and started treating it like the incredible creation that is ours alone. What if we woke up every morning and thanked our body for all it's efforts and encouraged it to be healthier by releasing extra weight. No more criticizing. Express love and appreciation for the body. Encourage it. Appreciate it. Trade hate for love and act like you mean it by your food choices and activities. I wonder what would happen then?

A new day

I'm almost sorry I bought Bob now. I didn't lose a pound the month of October. Yet I didn't do anything differently. In the past I would give up saying this doesn't work and begin eating my old ways again. But I am happy with what I eat now and there is nothing to rebel about. I eat whatever I'm hungry for.

I am truly beginning to trust my body. It will shed weight when it is ready. Anyway I have gone down three pants sizes and that is proof enough for me.

Sometimes I think about being a size ten again, and that would be nice. Also so much easier on my body. But I'll see how I feel and what nature has to say about that in the months and years to come.

A new day

Lately I've been crocheting a lot of scarves and hats for the homeless and it feels like exactly what I'm supposed to be doing. Up until a week or two ago I felt like it was a pretty menial pursuit but I no longer feel that way because of a movie I remember seeing several years ago. It was *Ghandi* and was the story of his life. In his later years he would sit on the ground with a wheel laying flat in front of him that was used to spin fiber into thread. I can still picture that. It made me realize that what I am doing is similar (though I certainly can't compare myself to Ghandi). But when I crochet I am happy and my thoughts tend to clear away the clouds. I suspect it was the same for him.

A new day

Tonight I had an open face toasted cheese sandwich and half a pear. I'm happy. And though I still have no appetite for pastry and pasta, I am still totally responsible for staying aware when I eat and that means only eating when I'm hungry. I know I ate more mixed nuts than I needed the other day.

A new day

Once again, I wish I hadn't bought Bob, except my curiosity gets the best of me. I have to stay away from him or I could start to feel sorry for myself.

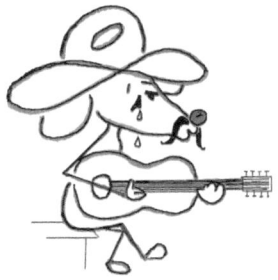

Yah want me to sing yah a sad song on my git box?

The body just isn't ready to shed pounds right now, so I think I'll put Bob in the man cave. I don't think I need to make any adjustments with food. I'll just go my merry way. Glad I don't have a compulsion to measure myself all the time, in fact I haven't done that at all. My undies are telling the story though because they are doing some serious draping.

A new day

There continues to be nothing I want to rebel against. I am enjoying my food and I feel good.

A new day

I've lost three pounds this week. The wall finally came down. Ah, the mysteries of the body. How long has it been since I was that other person?

Over eight months, and some good habits have become instilled in me I'm noticing when I start to think negatively and I'm able to stop and stay conscious while eating. Those things are pretty automatic now. Life is good and it just keeps getting better and better, and I am grateful.

A new day

Ouch. I have a black eye . . . literally. While taking a walk with the family, I tripped on the sidewalk and took a header. Didn't hurt much but boy do I look funny. It is really big and black.

So since I take responsibility with what happens in my life, it makes me look back at the thoughts I've generated lately. I have to admit I left the door open for some lousy thoughts and I have to think they were doing their generating job. I know better.

Negative thoughts are expensive but sometimes I slip up. Ah well. I'll do better in the future.

A new day

I am thrilled with Bob's number today and thinking that I haven't weighed this little since the 1980's. Wow! I still have a ways to go but it's a so what. I've learned that the longer you wear the extra weight the slower it's going to come off. That makes sense to me.

Staying conscious was the hard part for quite a while but habits have formed and pushing away food I don't want is second nature to me now. There are two foods I really miss, tomatoes and peaches, but that's because the local growers can't grow them in the winter. So I'll just have to wait for them.

A new day

My kids remarked that I walk faster now. I didn't realize it before but it's true, and I must have had a hard time hauling around the extra weight that is now gone.

A new day

I scared myself yesterday. I made biscotti to give as gifts for Christmas. Unhappily when I sliced it up it just crumbled. I had a huge heap of sweet pieces of pastry that were totally unsuitable as gifts. I began to slip into the old habit of eating what I knew I couldn't use. It was the old human garbage disposal habit sneaking up on me. Wow, I didn't know that was still lurking in my subconscious. Fortunately the alarms went off in my head and I sadly watched expensive ingredients gurgle down the disposal. Better it than me.

A new day

Christmas time, and I continue baking goodies for others. They're tasty but I still have no real desire to eat them. So different from Christmases past.

I've seen men on television lose 20-30 pounds in one week. But I am happy with my weight loss and I only exercise 20 minutes every day instead of 4-8 hours.

Not once in all this time have I denied myself anything I've felt hungry for. Of course paying attention to what my body is telling me has a lot to do with that. I enjoy the dried soups I get at the health food store. Pretty much no unidentifiable ingredients in them. But that's about it when I'm not in the produce section of the market. I am happy eating real food. I can remember buying bread at the store that lasted forever in the fridge. What in the world was in those loaves?

A new day

Oh boy. Christmas day I found myself alone with a bowl of guacamole sitting on the table. The family had left to go skiing. Okay. Okay. I scooped it up like there was no tomorrow. Did I stay conscious to that fact? Nooooo. And did my stomach let me know how it felt about that? Yessss. I spent a good deal of the afternoon with my head over the toilet. And when I barf it sounds like the mating call of a kimono dragon. It's not pretty. Anyway I am sadder but wiser today. It was a good lesson.

A new day and year, 2013

I went to an evening get together last night. There were all sorts of goodies to eat. I'm not a pizza lover but I tried a little of it plus a potato skin and a deviled egg. At the end of the evening I noticed something that struck me strange. On my plate I had left most of the pizza. I would have never done that in the past and I was happy with myself. It seems a conscious decision to only eat what I need no longer requires much thought. I don't even have to finish off things that taste extra good to me anymore.

Sanity came into my life and I now see food like a normal person. Thank goodness for the Get Out Of Jail Now card I pulled out of my back pocket. Life is good and it just keeps getting better and better.

A new day

Laid in bed and did an audit on what I am eating these days. I eat locally grown whenever possible, and during the winter when that isn't available I eat organic produce. The local grocery store is doing a pretty good job of stocking the shelves with locally grown and organic foods.

For me pasta and pastry is a thing of the past although it's okay occasionally. Never cook it for myself though. Fast food is a thing of the past too. All the grease, chemicals and salt just don't sound good to me.

Now and then my sweet tooth wants attention and I find a little box of raisins or a half piece of fruit is perfect, they are sweet and healthy. I only eat bread from the bakery where I know the ingredients don't come from a lab. That old commercial with the phrase "Better Living Through Chemistry" is fine but not on my plate.

A new day

Change has been so easy for me with this diet. I'm glad I included that word easy, in my affirmations. I really think that's an important key. It still seems hard to change other issues that crop up though. Right now I can think of a few things that need a change of attitude. Drat, I thought maybe I'd handled most of that stuff.

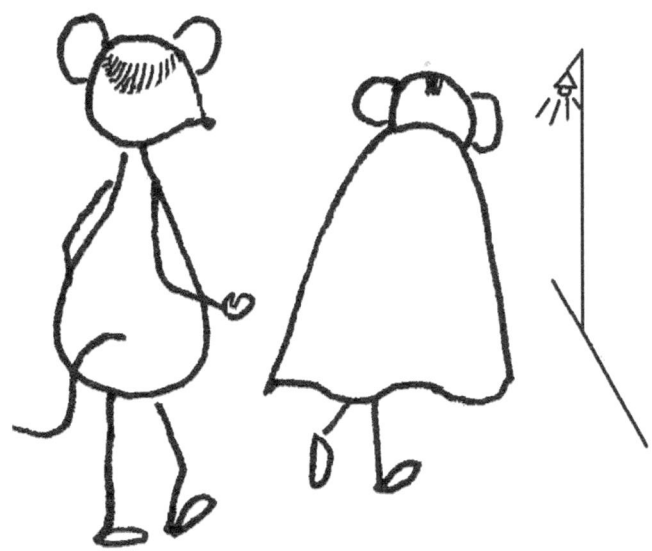

Jack: You don't look good Vammy. Draw some blood last night that didn't agree?

Vammy: For sure. Tell Velvita to lay off the junk food. I can't handle all those chemicals.

Jack: Maybe it's time you gave up the business Vammy.

Vammy: What? And give up perks like my comfy coffin?

Jack: Well, it's up to you. But for me I'll take a bed I can stretch out in, drink my chocolate almond coffee and read the funnies.

Vammy: Stretch out?! Chocolate almond coffee?!! Funnies?!!! Sigh.

A new day

With the holidays past and the Christmas movies finally over the programs telling you how to lose weight run rampant. Some ideas make sense to me. Others, not so much.

I know fad diets don't work. In fact all diets are doomed to fail in time. They just work against human nature. We are meant to enjoy eating, but our taste buds are so far off track these days. Fast foods taste good but the vast majority of it isn't good for the body.

A new day

I still feel there are other reasons for being overweight that are seldom mentioned, and the main one is the core belief we have about ourselves and negative thinking from the past that accompanies it.

Until we heal and dump the negative feelings like criticism, resentment, fear of failure and guilt we will continue to run afoul of food. We need to face them down once and for all. The sorrow has to come out, or at least it did for me. And positive thinking has to take its place.

A new day

How lucky I am to be able to stay in and cook up some beef soup in the crock pot while it snows outside. The weather also made me pensive, and I think back to when I was a kid and what dinner was like. My family always had a pleasant dinner experience. The only thing I hated was some of the food. I remember hiding boiled carrots under my seat cushion. We all looked forward to dessert since my mom was a great baker. "No dessert till you clean your plate", I would hear. I'd do anything for some of that chocolate banana devil's food cake. It was heaven.

A new day

I've come to the conclusion that sugar was just about the last thing my body wanted to process. I suspect it all turned to fat in my system. And I remember how painful it was for me to be a fat kid and how so many kids are experiencing that these days.

In a perfect world we'd have all overweight kids retaught to listen to their stomach and never eat dessert directly after dinner. If I had my way they would spend at least fifteen minutes eating the main course. Then take ten minutes to socialize at the table either simply talking or playing some sort of simple game, something to take their minds off food. At the end of that time they could check in with their stomach and feel whether it needed more food or not and then have a dessert, preferably fruit.

Dessert would also be a good time to enforce slow eating, and to learn to really enjoy what's going down rather than just gobbling something sweet. Most of us have messed up eating habits, and it's sad to pass that on to kids.

A new day

It's a good thing I'm learning patience with this lifestyle. Yesterday a new electronic device I'd ordered arrived. Within a couple hours it stopped working. Have to return it to the maker. Okay, okay it was probably my fault for pushing too many wrong buttons. Ah well, they will send me a new one in a few days.

I haven't lost a pound in three weeks but I'm not surprised or upset. The body knows when the time is right and I'm okay with that after all these months. I trust it and myself.

A new day

Well, not so much on the trust thing today. I trust the wisdom of my body but now I'm wondering if I'm I doing something wrong. There is still no reason to change what I eat, but maybe I'm eating too much. Well, all I can do is my best. I know the weight I'm carrying around now has been there for 20 or 30 years. Maybe it's just a little too comfortable.

A new day

Yesterday afternoon I was totally engrossed watching an interesting DVD. I had the whim to go get on my treadmill and exercise. I thought, okay, that's a good idea. I'll do it as soon as I finish the DVD. My whim would have none of it. It kept going through my mind to go exercise. Finally after about ten minutes of that I turned off the half done

DVD and went to the treadmill. I don't know how long I was on it but it felt wonderful. I'm going to do that every afternoon from now on along with my morning exercise.

I learned two things from this, changing my attitude about exercise does wonders and a whim or a notion is what I call the angels pushing me. Sometimes angels nudge, sometimes push and other times shove and I know all are worth our attention.

A new day

I woke up this morning not feeling as happy as usual and decided it was time to get out my mental bug spray and find out what's going on. And I soon did. Something I said to my daughter was bothering me. I'd said something I now wish I hadn't. Drat. It is disappointing to be reminded that I'm still only human. Ah well, it just means there is more learning to do.

I wouldn't mind having an egg and hash browns this morning for breakfast but I'm out of eggs until I go to the ranch market tomorrow. Then I remembered I have stewed blackberries in the refrigerator. Yeah!

A new day

I hadn't lost a pound since Christmas Eve but today one finally let go. Yeah!

I've thought a lot about when I was gaining and losing the most weight through my lifetime. It's true that emotions play a big part especially the negative ones we ignore or hardly are aware of. They bug us and then get permanently under our skin in the form of fat, alcohol or another form of addiction. They're like some nasty little insect.

There have been times without number that I ate something when I wasn't hungry. For me I was self medicating sorrow and loneliness with food. It brings tears to my eyes remembering how often I did that. There was sorrow with the divorce and the great life style my kids and I left behind, and worse was they only had a father around occasionally. It broke my heart, and weight became a constant struggle.

A new day

I'm reading a book titled *Fast Food Nation* by Eric Schlosser. It's been around several years. Do you know why a burger and fries taste good? It's not because of the ingredients you see. It's due to all the chemicals in them made in a New Jersey laboratory. It makes me wonder if all those chemicals have any negative lasting effect on the human body. What happens to us after consuming them for many years? Also could they, like cigarettes, become habit forming? What effect do they have on kids? If you think banks and Wall St. have been unethical just check out the fast food industry. You might want to check out who the industry contributes to at election time too.

A new day

I've been meditating again for the past few weeks. Deepak Chopra and my daughter helped me get a clearer understanding of meditation. The way I see it now is it's like an electrical outlet and just sits there on the wall waiting. But recharge your laptop with it and all sorts of nifty things are available to you. That's how it is with meditation. Plug in once a day and let it do its magic in the form of ideas and whims at a later time. Anyway that's how it is for me.

I also spend time each morning thinking about all I'm grateful for, and send love and blessings to everyone I can think of. Science is beginning to say we rewire our brains when we do stuff like that and I strongly suspect it's true.

A new day

They say the hardest thing about losing weight is keeping it off. I see where that makes sense if you are doing some crazy diet that denies you eating some of the things you love or are hungry for. But I never deny myself anything so what will happen? It will be quite a while before I need to stop losing weight so I'm not going to worry about it. It's nearly a year that I've been doing food this way and I never would have thought this weight loss could happen, especially at my age.

A new day

I wonder from time to time why my "diet" is taking so long, and I've realized three reasons for it. One, I asked for an easy, natural, happy, and healthy way to lose weight. I found that and it is slower than the crazy diets but it is sure.

The second is I've had lessons to learn along the way like trust and patience that also takes some time. And the third thing is I never really owned the philosophy behind the belief system the universe is supporting me. I've acknowledged it and done my best to practice it but it's never quite been mine.

It's like I've had it on layaway all my life. Now it's no longer something I intellectually accept but something I own. I've taken it home and realize it's this enormous gift of letting go of negative energy and falling in love with myself. Wow. Love that Get Out Of Jail Now card. I have to tell you that card rocks!

A new day

Today I did something I never thought I'd do. I put Bob away in his man cave indefinitely. I read somewhere that if you are too invested in results, resolutions will get stopped up. So I don't know when I'll see Bob again.

I've decided to let go of what I want and just go about the business of being sane and conscious about food. I've learned to trust my body's wisdom over time and I loved seeing those pounds disappear. But maybe I need to just let go of that for now. I'll see how I feel about it as time goes on.

A new day

I've decided to do my best to let go of all expectations regarding weight. I know a person needs clarity about what they want, but for me, it's better if I don't define that desire too much. I like to control the future if I think I can find a way to get away with it. But often my way has gotten me and others into trouble. Besides, if I just relax things work out better than I dreamed they ever would.

A new day

I went dumpster diving this morning figuratively speaking. I was knee deep in crud like painful experiences that I thought I'd discarded years ago.

I knew that this could hold up any good that was going to come into my life and it was time to forgive my ex and myself once again.

I also thought about that pesky Bob. I have to say I don't miss him. Anyway, my undies say it pretty clearly. Thelma and Louise need a smaller size now.

A new day

I've been very pensive lately. This morning I was thinking about our power of choice.

It's easy for me to understand why dieting was such a pain in the past. There were constant choices to make every waking moment of the day. Do I choose to "behave" or am I going to eat those cookies? I loved chocolate chip cookies so I ate them, usually all of them that were visible to me.

Out of sight, out of mind worked for me sometimes but not always. It was much easier to give up. Besides, all that sugar made me feel better while it was going down. And of course there was that core belief that said I was the consummate failure.

It wasn't until I faced myself in the mirror that day the old belief system could be kicked out of my life and the true power of choice restored. Thank goodness my choices were still available when it came to choosing between positive and negative thinking.

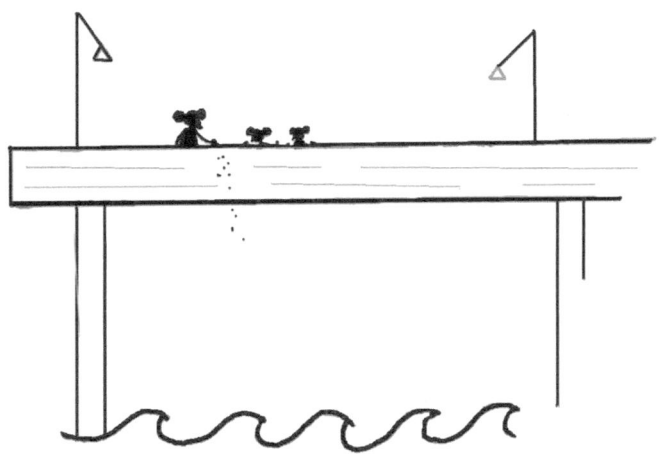

Cam: What are you going to do with all that salt Granddad?

Jack: I'm having a thanksgiving. I'm grateful for all my freedoms, my good health and cheese makers everywhere.

Cole: How come you throw a pinch of salt in the water with each thank you?

Jack: Makes it more real to me. I get to see my gratitude dissolve into the universe. I do the same thing with problems. It helps me to see myself letting go. Works great.

Cam: Boy, you must have a lot of gratitude and problems. We swam in this water last summer and it's got a lotta salt in it.

My friends and I did this at the Huntington Beach Pier. It really does help.

A new day

Gradually I am learning to trust myself when it comes to food. A new lifestyle has definitely set in. I couldn't imagine doing without bread in the past and now it's no longer important to me. I still like it but has fallen into the same slot as pastries, pasta, pop and processed foods. They all taste good to me but I live very happily without them. I eat as much organic food as possible and am happy about that. I still love beef and chicken, but now I wouldn't think of buying anything that wasn't grass fed, free range and chemical free.

A new day

I've discovered something that has helped me through the hard part of meditation, clearing the mind. I picture myself holding a broom and I'm sweeping out a room. I feel the rhythm of sweeping and I hear the bristles brushing across the floor. I sweep out all thoughts to make room for divine intelligence. It is very, very tranquilizing. In fact I call it my tranquilizer broom.

I'm not exceedingly fond of sweeping in everyday life, but I felt I could do this all day, and this morning I lifted my head while sweeping to see what the room looked like. I saw clearly that it was an empty classroom, no furniture, and nothing on the walls. And I was getting it ready. Meditation usually comes naturally now. Life is good and it just keeps getting better and better.

A new day

Well, not so much but it's okay. This morning I met with Bob (yes, he is out of the man cave again) to see that I had gained a pound. No big deal except that today is February 8 and I had only lost one pound since Christmas Day. Ugh. Have I been doing food differently? I don't think so. Did I get the same amount of exercise? No. I'd increased my daily exercises from fifteen minutes in the morning to a half hour and fifteen minutes in the afternoon. I have no idea what's going on. I do know there remains to be no reason to walk away. I am happy with my meals and since I decided to change my attitude about the treadmill, I actually find it to be like an old friend to me. Who knew? I trust that if there is something else that needs to be done by me, it will come to me. One happy thing I noticed today. My pants are getting too big. I need a size smaller again. That will make me four sizes smaller. Sounds good to me. And I see I better change my thinking about weight loss now.

A new day

This morning I watched *Gary Zukav* on television and he said something that struck me. He said everything we do in life is either based on love or fear. I knew I was in fear. I was afraid I wasn't in control of my body. I was afraid the pounds would just stop rolling off. I was afraid to look at the scales. I was afraid I would always feel this way.

Then I remembered something I already knew. When a feeling like that comes up, stop and take a look at it and don't run away and ignore it. For me I realize I am not in control, and I don't like that. Hey Zukav, hand me the Kleenex.

A new day

I realized something in the last days. It's obviously none of my business what is going on inside my body. Stuff happens in there constantly that I have absolutely no knowledge of and never will. I do know that if I am following my optimum way of doing food and by thinking right I can rest easy.

A new day

Measuring my weight loss against someone that is 50 or younger doesn't make sense. My lifestyle is something of an experiment now. I don't know any healthy person over 65 who has had a lifelong struggle with weight and lost a significant amount in their senior years. Interesting.

A new day

Ouch. I am struggling to keep my thinking in check. Am I ever going to lose more weight? Maybe I'm too old or I've just been wearing this fat too long. I don't know, but it makes me want to cry. Again I've put Bob away. I feel I've lost my way.

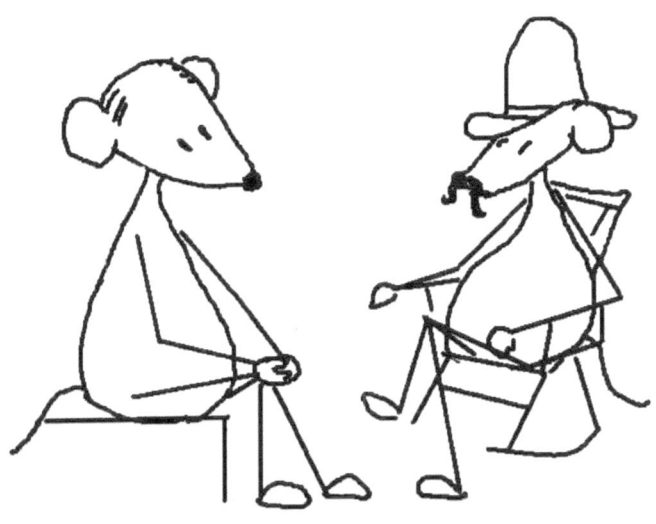

Jack: When did you learn to drive Uncle Smokey?

Smokey Cheddar: Well, let's see now. I was about eleven and out at the ranch. I drove all over the place out there. Then when I was about fifteen Aunt Maude asked me if I could drive her back East. I said sure and I even read the rule book before we left. I didn't hit nothin' either till we got to Illinois.

I sometimes feel like I've been driving around in Illinois.

A new day

It turns out that so far the hardest lesson I've had to learn on this "diet" is giving up my expectations and control. I continue to do the three things that I think need to be done by me: eat with sanity, stay conscious, exercise and think positive. Well, not today with that last one. I feel some deep disappointment right now. Expectations and control have always been a part of my life. Can I really dump them?

A new day

It is clear to me now that trust is another issue. Intellectually I know what the truth is for me, but as far as trust that's something I've never really owned. For me, it's still in layaway and I haven't taken it home yet. In the past I was so disappointed with myself and now I'm scared that will happen again. I understand I don't have to feel that way anymore, but I do. Especially when I look at Bob and he doesn't budge. It all just brings me to my knees.

This too will pass.

A new day

I woke this morning still trying to "get it". I see now that faith and trust are not the bedrock of the equation I'm looking for, it's the energy I supply. Then faith and trust are automatic. It's really simple. Just stick with the feelings that make me happy, glad, joyous, loving, tolerant and grateful, and discard the things that make me feel bad. Staying conscious and paying attention when the angels are pushing, that's important. And from there I need to keep my busy little fingers out of the game.

In other words don't try to control the outcome. That part is none of our business. My job is just to do my best.

I've found the currency to pull these concepts out of layaway and take them home. They belong to me now. Weight is not so much the issue as is the energy I put out in the form of thoughts and actions.

A new day

I suspect that everything in the universe has energy, and for sure our thoughts. I don't think the universe forgets either. So it is totally important to keep our thoughts in a positive mode. We're human so we mess up sometimes. But that can be corrected and the sooner the better. I am so thankful I was born into a family of happy people. They made mistakes too, but oh, how many positive seeds they planted for me.

A new day

My mind is busy before I get out of bed in the morning. I mentioned previously that I thought it would be a good idea to praise our bodies instead of always being so critical of them. Now I'm thinking we need to adopt the same attitude with our body that we have for our old friends. We love and care about them. They feel the love we give them and it is reflected back to us. I think our body needs that kind of loving attitude from us too.

A new day

I have to be honest. The jury is still out for me as far as meditation goes. I still think it's a lovely place to be but I am clueless what it is generating. I did the meditation challenge with Oprah and Deepak Chopra and thought it was wonderful. But I come out with the same thought, why am I doing this? I don't feel or see any results.

I am very pragmatic at times, or maybe I'm just plain skeptical. But if I don't see results or feel something is working for me it seems time to shelve it. And that's what I'm going to do for now. As I've said before, people I respect meditate. Maybe I'm doing it wrong or my expectations are out of line.

A new day

Spinach salad planned for dinner tonight. I think my taste buds are growing more discerning. I bought my favorite sub for lunch today but I have to say it no longer tasted as good is it did in the past. The restaurants veggies were very tired. I guess there is nothing like homemade food.

A new day

Yesterday I talked to my son in Phoenix. He is faced with a rather difficult choice. He has thought a lot about moving here to Durango to be around family and start a business of his own. But he's concerned with the choice of giving up all the perks with his present job like a generous number of paid days off, medical insurance and a nice steady pay check. That is hard to leave behind, and I don't know what he'll choose to do. He is very careful with money. (There had to be one of us in the family.)

A new day

All winter I've had a runny nose. How can that be? The trees are bare and the ground is covered in snow. I can't blame it on allergies. I think it must have something to do with my thought patterns. I did a little more thinking and realized I'm still scared I'm not going to lose any more weight. I have a long history of giving up on diets. Of course this isn't really a diet, but it does involve shedding extra weight. My fears about weight were getting the best of me and the energy I was putting out was not good even though I'm meditating again. I have to say I cried off and on for about two weeks. Then one day it started. These concepts that had been in layaway most of my life I realized I owned now and I could take them home.

It occurred to me I wasn't being specific enough with my words when I do my devotionals every morning. I wasn't speaking my word for anything. The time was spent in gratitude and sending love and healing to everyone I could think of, which I still do. But when I said "Thank you for the weight loss" it seems the universe simply said "You're welcome" and nothing happened beyond that.

This sounds weird but I think my prayers were too lady like. By that I mean I was doing what we women are often scripted to do, be nice, mind our manners by saying thank you and dispensing love. This morning I happened to see Pastor Olsteen on television. He said to dream big and pray boldly. That really struck a chord with me. I'm going to start asking for what I want in a clear, concise way along with the love and gratitude. I think I've been missing the boat.

A new day

I've wanted to retrieve Bob again and weigh myself. But my relationship with him is still tenuous, besides I want to wait until the first year anniversary of this new life which will come in a few days.

I've been using the treadmill every afternoon for fifteen minutes. But yesterday I found a music channel on television that I like. I danced to the music for fifteen minutes and got an even better workout than on the treadmill. I think that's what I'll do in the afternoons from now on and increase the time.

A new day

Results of this lifestyle showed up at the doctor's office the other day after annual lab results. She was quite shocked how much the numbers had improved. It seems the body really does respond to love and appreciation. I wonder what all goes on in there sometimes.

A new day

Today is the one year mark for my new life and I decided to take Bob out of his man cave and get a feel of what our relationship is like these days. I found out. It is very much like the relationship that my great, great grandparents had. In their later years she lived in town and he lived out in the country. He'd visit her once in awhile, and we can draw our own conclusions about that. Anyway, that's how it is with Bob. I am at peace with him now, especially since I am no longer compulsive about him. We'll probably get together again sometime but it's not important to know when. I guess I just don't need him anymore.

The weight loss slowed down these past few months. I realize my negative thinking and frustration with Bob didn't help at all, and I suspect the weight loss will improve a bit now that I've cleaned up my attitude.

A new day

I've learned some great lessons in the past year. Concepts I bought years ago were finally ready to come out of layaway and bring home. I own them now. It is strange how we can totally stick with our beliefs for years on end yet don't own them. It's when we get it in our gut and live it that they are truly ours.

A new day

I went to the local market today with a few things on my list. One was peanut butter. I studied most of the jars on the shelf, and all had mystery ingredients I couldn't pronounce or understand why they were added. I know now it's to make the peanuts go farther, and last longer.

Then one jar caught my attention. But I couldn't find any ingredients listed. Finally I spotted the list in a tiny corner, and it had one thing on the ingredients list: peanuts. Wow, who would have thought of it! Maybe the food companies are getting the idea.

A new day

Have you ever noticed how hard asphalt is. You'd have to take a hammer and chisel to break it up. But let rain or snow sit on it for awhile and asphalt just dissolves. That's how cola acts with your bones. Bones are made to last a lifetime but keep drinking pop and bones will weaken and dissolve too.

A new day

I wish the growers would stop growing strawberries with steroids or whatever it is that makes them so big. They have so little flavor. Don't they think we notice?

There is just nothing like local growers. James Ranch here in Durango grows the most amazing vegetables. My favorites are the heirloom tomatoes. How I wish they had a longer season. And the crazy carrots they grow are so good and also quite funny looking. They aren't just orange but purple and blond, short, tall, lumpy and twisted. And the ranch fresh eggs harvested are wonderful. By the way, their hens aren't fed soy anymore because they got aggressive when eating it. (I wonder if soy affects humans in a negative way.) Anyway the hens are allowed to act like chickens. They peck for worms in the pasture and then return to their own mobile home in the evening. What a life.

I've never had a Georgia peach but the peaches grown in Colorado are so sweet and flavorful, and when you bite into one the juice runs down to your elbow. Happily they will be ripe soon.

A new day

I wonder about hybrid veggies and fruit sometimes. Actually I don't think being hybrid is a bad thing. Look at humans. Most of us are quite a mix and I are pretty healthy. What I don't like are the chemicals added to so many things. Read the ingredients on the labels.

And if you don't have the time to do that, at least take note whether there is a long list. If there is, the product is probably stuffed with chemicals and preservatives created in New Jersey.

A new day

This morning my mind said something like "What are you thinking eating so much cheese. It was right. Some of my choices have been a little out of line. Thank goodness for the sanity factor that's now in my head.

A new day

I continue to correct my course like a torpedo. Although I am happy with my body I still know that it would have an easier time of it if there was less weight to haul around. And since weight loss has been sluggish, I'm looking around to see what else I can do. Certainly I won't be counting calories or carbs or fat grams. That's over.

A new day

This morning I thought more about staying conscious with my choices. I know I'm eating the right amount to lose weight easily and naturally in a happy, healthy way. Food choices are pretty easy for me now yet I still look back and wonder about the amounts I eat. I know I forget to stay conscious about that sometimes. I'm clear about my intentions, but I seem to forget them when sitting down to a meal sometimes.

It's a lot like using shopping bags. I bought the bags about five years ago to use at the grocery store instead of using their plastic bags. At first I'd forget to put them in the car, then I had them in the car but often forgot to take them into the store. But in the past couple of years there has been no problem getting them into the store. It's a habit.

I think it's that way with the amounts of food I eat. Even after more than a year, I need to stay conscious. It isn't a habit yet. I wonder about these people who say it takes three weeks to form a habit. Who are they talking to?

A new day

It seems cheese has gone the way of pastry. I still like it but it isn't at all important to me. I think I had it once in the past week. I love my new found sanity. It works so well.

PART III

My Diet Plan

Books that talk about diets always include a diet plan. So I'll tell you my plan. I plan to enjoy food as much as possible, and here is a list of my favorite meals. I'm not telling you what to eat, I just want to give you an idea what works for me.

<u>Breakfast</u>

I don't like breakfast even when I'm hungry. Here is what I eat to fill the void.

Half a bagel with butter or peanut butter or both.

Soft boiled egg spread over toast.

I like these two breakfasts because there is almost no clean up involved.

Cereal from health food store with non fat dry milk, raspberries previously stewed in sugar and a handful of walnuts.

Lunch

Egg salad using two eggs and greens

Subway's spicy Italian foot long sub. I eat half the foot long after tearing off the top half of the bread. I save the bread for the birds and eat the other half of the filling as an antipasto salad after adding greens. I have that for dinner or lunch the next day.

Quasadilla with one tortilla from health food store, filled with cheese, tomato and onion.

Dinner

Grass fed chuck roast I cook in the crock pot with a packet of roast seasoning. I split it up and freeze what I'm not going to use right away. I like it with barbeque sauce in a bun, or with oven roasted veggies or in chili.

Tostado. I think I could eat Mexican food seven days a week.

Big green salad with everything on it: croutons, avocado, green onions, olives or whatever sounds good.

Tomato soup from the health food store and parmesan "cookies". (Make little piles of shredded parmesan on a baking sheet. Bake for seven minutes in a 400 degree oven.) Great combo.

Dessert

Yogurt with stewed fruit and walnuts.

Fruit.

Snacks

Fresh fruit with cheese or walnuts. I also buy coconut covered dates at the health food store. They are delicious and one of them keeps my stomach happy for a couple hours.

Drinks

Hot or cold lemonade

Lipton's tea with pomegranate and cranberry. I like it with a little honey.

Hot nonfat milk with honey and vanilla.

I drink a glass of red or white wine every evening before dinner.

On a cold snowy morning there is nothing like a cup of hot chocolate. I make it with nonfat dry milk, unsweetened cocoa, sugar and, okay, a shot of brandy. Yum!

PART IV

The Last Word

I spent most of my life in Southern California. In the summer it seemed like everyone headed for the beach in the morning. Some went down Beach Blvd., others took Harbor and others went through Laguna Canyon, and we all got to the beach. The point is everyone has their own way. This journal reflects the way I've followed. We all don't choose the same way and I honor that. Of course I have my opinions. I think some ways are pretty roundabout and others have too many stop lights, but that's just my opinion. Sooner or later we all get to the beach.

It's the same idea with words and names. Some people use the word God. I like the word universe. But we're still all going to the beach so I'm okay with letting go of semantics.

I'm back meditating again. I still wonder if I'm practicing it effectively. When I meditate I feel like I'm wandering around in the dark and I don't know why. I guess we Americans are still beginners at this. Sometimes I fall asleep. I've learned one thing about it. I don't rush it. If I have a number of things whizzing around in my mind like phone calls I need to make, I do my best to take care of those things before I sit down to meditate. It makes it easier to clear my mind. I've also learned to have clear intentions before I begin. Usually that is to clear the way for guidance.

I suspect that it's like learning to play a musical instrument. Practice makes perfect and a person doesn't master it right away. I believe that it does affect our lives because my whims, dreams and concerns seem to be resolved in short order. Larger issues have taken more time. I also sleep much better now that I meditate.

I see now that this book isn't as much about weight or about what I eat as it is about the way I think and the emotional baggage I had hauled around. In the past I was off course in the way I thought and felt and that had to do with being overweight. I had to let go of the energy on sadness and fear and take responsibility for the power that I have inside. I don't want to run away from that power any more by eating too much, spending too much or just being too busy to notice what feelings are telling us.

I cherish that day last year when I told my daughter I planned to do my best to stay away from negative thinking. There is no doubt in my mind that was what blew away old attitudes. And the mirror work cinched it. I can't say how much weight I've lost since I didn't have a scale when this first started but I can say I am down four pant sizes.

I'm grateful that I changed my thinking about exercise too. By the way, a great way to start exercising is to find a music channel on your TV and dance. The time goes fast and you'll work up a sweat. Plus, it doesn't cost anything and you can do it in your jammies if you want to.

I'm also thankful for finally owning the idea that every thought I have is pure energy and is continually creating my health and future circumstances. I read somewhere that our bodies are constantly eavesdropping on our thoughts and feelings. I believe that's true.

The way I interpret universe now is the energy that we are all born with and live with is eternal. This is probably bizarre to many people but I think when we die our energy remains totally intact and we go back to being part of the universe as pure energy. That also clarifies the phrase we hear that we are all one. That seems logical to me now because we all are sharing the same energy and probably passing it around like I'm doing here. And when we pray or meditate souls that are now in the form of pure energy come and guide us.

You can decide for yourself what to think. I always like to say, when you're reading or listening to others beliefs don't leave your brains at the Table Of Contents or in the parking lot. Think for yourself.

For the first time in my life I trust myself, my body and the universe. I am at peace with the way I do food, exercise and with my thinking. Don't get me wrong. Sometimes I mess up with my thoughts. That doesn't hang around now. In the past those thoughts would torment me for weeks, months and even years.

I have to laugh at myself when I think back at my relationship with Bob. Talk about screwed up thoughts and attitudes! That game is over. Bob and I get together now and then but I no longer fight with him since I don't need his approval any more. We are more like old friends with a very long history.

I expect more weight loss eventually and that will be great. But the big win is not the number on the scales but, rather the fact that after all these years I've made peace with my body and I accept the power within. I love that. It's like my relationship with Bob. We are friends now and when we mess up we are quick to forgive.

Life is good and it just keeps getting better and better.

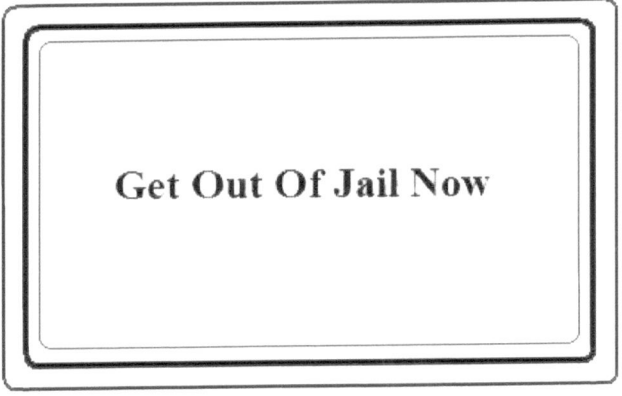

Get Out Of Jail Now

Visit the website at www.dietingwithdena.com

Some Of My Favorite Teachers

Louise Hay

"How To Heal Your Life", that's the book that began changing my life. She has written a lot of other books. Check out her web site.

Deepak Chopra

He appears on the OWN network often, and I loved his meditation class. He's written numerous books. Check out his web site.

Gary Zukav

He also appears with Oprah pretty often and has several books out. Amazon carries all of these favorites of mine.

Carolyn Myss

Appears on Oprah's shows now and then and has also written several books.

<u>Florence Schinn</u>

Her book *"The Game Of Life And How To Play It"* was written in the 1920's and is still totally relevant.

Rhonda Byrne
"The Secret"

This comes in a book and DVD. I have both.

Oprah Winfrey's OWN network brings us many wonderful teacher on Sundays.